The YOGA of HEALTHY NUTRITION

Doctor Lynn Wylnn

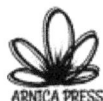

ARNICA PRESS

I0039461

The material contained in this book has been written for informational purposes and is not intended as a substitute for medical advice, nor is it intended to diagnose, treat, cure, or prevent disease. If you have a medical issue or illness, consult a qualified physician.

Published by ARNICA PRESS

www.ArnicaPress.com

ARNICA PRESS

Printed in the United States of America.

ISBN: 978-1-955354-21-9

The YOGA of HEALTHY NUTRITION

Doctor LYNN WYLNN

BOOK ONE

BY DOCTOR LYNN WYLNN

THE SOUL WALKING SERIES:

HOW TO MASTER KARMA

HOW TO PROSPER WITH A PURPOSE

HOW TO MASTER VITALITY

NATURALLY SEXY AND HEALTHY

RECIPES FOR HEALTH, SEX, HAPPINESS AND LOVE

THE NATUROPATHIC WELLNESS SERIES:

THE YOGA OF HEALTHY NUTRITION

NATUROPATHIC RECIPES

A NATUROPATHIC APPROACH TO THE ANCIENT PATH OF

Anna- Maya-Kosha-Yoga

THE ESSENCE OF FOOD AND DIET

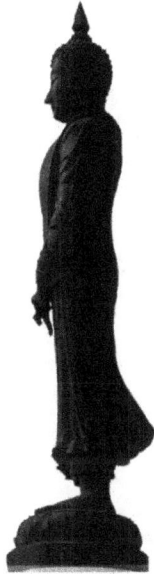

To my children who were my recipe testers
and all my students and clients who faithfully followed my advice —
honor your health. It is truly your wealth.

TABLE OF CONTENTS

INTRODUCTION

Anna- Maya- Kosha is the branch of yoga dedicated to conscious eating. It promotes the principles of inspecting what and how we eat, for the essence of food has a direct effect upon our physical, mental and soulful being. Yoga is an all-inclusive discipline, ignoring no aspect of human existence, which includes our diets.

Thousands of years ago yogis understood that our bodies and our minds are functional units that reflect the very state of our being. Honoring the body-mind with nutritious life-giving food brings about balance and health. The primary journey of yoga is spiritual, which requires clarity and balance, and it is well understood that when the body-mind is in a state of agitation due to a poor diet, clarity and balance cannot be found. We often look at poor diet, lack of exercise, and self neglect as the causative factors in disease and energy imbalance. However, these are really a reflection of our own inner inability to treat the underlying cause, which is not to simply attempt to cure a disease, but to strive to return us to a state of healthy balance in body, mind and soul. The spiritual path is a conscious approach with a reverence for all of life, which includes the state of our health body, mind and soul. Therefore, we should always seek to honor that which brings us health, vitality and joy.

Balance and vitality are the key concept of Anna-maya-kosha yoga. It is through the promotion of balance that, we should seek to find balance in all things and in all things finds balance. Balance is a reflection of the vitality and strength of the body-mind and this vitality comes about when we feed the vehicle of the soul with life giving nourishment. Health is a refection of a state of balance and vitality. We cannot find balance until we develop a change in attitude, and find peace of mind and inner happiness. This takes self-discipline which is the conscious choice to promote vitality and do no harm. It is about promoting the ideals of a long and healthy life, which means to consciously promote health rather than a focus on the eradication of disease.

The ideals of a long and healthy life means that we experience radiant health which includes physical vitality and adaptability, sexual vigor and response, mental acuity, anti-aging, love and compassion, harmonious relationships, happiness and wisdom. This is found through a state of balance, harmony and peace.

There is a growing recognition among healthcare providers that one of the most basic ways of ensuring the ideals of a healthy and long life is through proper diet combined with exercise. However, the obesity rate for Americans is on the rise, in part due to fast foods and lack of exercise. Anna-maya-kosha yoga teaches the consciousness of the impact of food on our total state of being. Combining the practice of Anna-maya-kosha yoga with asana (physical) work, and soulful meditation, an individual will find balance and harmony, and this will bring in its train health, happiness and wisdom.

This book will take you through the physical, mental and soulful journey of conscious choice making regarding your diet. It is not about eating a strict vegetarian diet, or following any prescribed diet plan. Anna-maya-kosha yoga is about awareness of the choices we make and how the choices reflect in our body-mind.

Anna-maya-kosha is a path of yoga. There are six major branches; the best understood is hatha, the asanas, or the physical poses and postures. Anna-maya-kosha yoga enhances the asana work.

The purpose of this book is to assist you in searching out the inner way through the awareness of what it means to live a harmonious and healthy life. Although it is a book about the yoga branch of eating, it is also a practical map for the conquest of the inner reflection of the soulful self that dwells within.

Therefore, it is hoped that through these pages you will find not only the philosophy of honoring the body-mind through the choice of diet, but also the deeper meaning that is hidden within the discipline of yoga.

Supposedly Buddha said that the first step to Nirvana is perfect health, and the way to attain it is to follow the eight-fold path, which is the prescription for ending all suffering. The first two paths are concerned with right seeing and right knowing, the next four steps have to do with right action, (karma yoga and Anna-maya-kosha-yoga), and the last two are concerned with right awareness and right contemplation, and describes the direct mystical experience of reality that is the ultimate goal. This path is found through the principles and branches of yoga, usually beginning with hatha. The asanas (poses and postures) are not simply a set of exercises, but meant to be practiced as one of the branches, combined with the other branches, leading to a spiritual way of life.

Many aspects of yoga have a Hindu flavor; however, the true practice of yoga is not about following a prescribed religion, or set of beliefs, but rather about discovering self-awareness through the experience.

Yoga therefore is a universal art, which grows when a person is dedicated to discovering a life of higher values and ideals.

Our modern-day western lifestyle is more complex than ever. It is clearly far more complex than the traditional society of India, (where yoga developed) and must be taken into account when we practice yoga here in the West. Lifestyles, attitudes and dietary habits are far different in traditional ancient societies. However, the West can gain tremendous benefits from the principles of yoga. Combining hatha (physical) yoga with Karma yoga, the path of transcending action, will enhance the spiritual process. Karma yoga seeks to break the vicious cycle of actions that lead to destruction and negativity and guides us towards the true purpose of our life's work which is to perform that service which benefits others, or better said, *find a need and fill it*. It can bring a sense of accomplishment, satisfaction, and balance to our work oriented western culture.

If we then add to these two branches, the yogic principle of eating, Anna-maya-kosha, we begin to practice the basic moral observance of inspecting what and how we feed the body-mind to ensure the optimum in health. For remember, the path to nirvana is the perfection of health, and no aspect of existence should be ignored. Yoga is all-inclusive and understanding this we should always strive to choose that which creates the greatest good and does the least harm.

It can be said of many books and philosophical disciplines, there may be within the context a message that may not be apparent on the surface. Suggested meanings and allegorical stories give birth to deep and mysterious secrets. In yoga it is often referred to as the occult, which simply means, that which is hidden from the average person. To discover the secret is simply to apply the discipline of conscious awareness. Anna-maya-kosha yoga is a discipline that will open the door to discovering the inner essence of a healthy and vital life.

Inside these pages is a prescribed set of steps that will lead towards experiencing the radiance of a healthy and balanced life. Following the path will not bring immediate gratification, for that is not the path of yoga. This is not about a "quick fix" but rather the long learning process of the attainment of wisdom. However, if you follow the path of Anna-maya-kosha-yoga, within 30 to 60 days you will begin to experience lightness, peacefulness, and a radiant vitality in your body, mind, and soul. This is the path of radiant health: seek balance in all things and in all things, you will find balance.

Namaste

I celebrate the place within where our souls will meet.

Doctor Lynn

PRANA-MAYA-KOSHA YOGA
~ THE CONCEPT OF LIFE ENERGY

To understand Anna-maya-kosha, which means the essence of food energy, we need to understand the concept of Prana – maya- kosha, which means the essence of energy. Prana is the vital link between physical body consciousness and astral consciousness, which is the consciousness of our emotions.

The life force that vitalizes everything in the universe is called Prana in Yogic healing. It is actually the energy of consciousness, responsible for the movement of all consciousness in the world. All systems of healing (even allopathic) use some form of prana. This is because prana is about vitality and balance. Vitality and balance are what brings about and maintains health. Naturopaths teach body-mind balance and integration to bring about and maintain health. Once achieved, we can get to the higher aspects of life, being the spiritual self. Prana actually comes from the Sanskrit word-meaning vital force. It is the basis of Ayer Veda, the traditional healing system of India.

Prana also relates to Yoga. Yoga is not just a system of exercise, or meditation but a way of working the subtle energies of the body and the mind through the force of prana. The breathing exercises associated with yoga are based upon an understanding of prana.

Natural health uses various substances such as food, herbs, oils, water, exercise and meditation as vehicles for prana. Depending upon our need for heat or cooling determines the substance used. Natural health systems also use acupuncture, bodywork, or pancha karma (Ayurvedic purification) to work on prana. Touch by itself is a form of prana as it communicates energy directly.

All disease, whether it is mental, or physical, reflects a breakdown of pranic energy. Depression, debility, sadness, or any other negative emotional state indicates pranic imbalance. Therefore, it is important to keep prana in healthy balance.

So, what is prana and where does it come from? And what does it have to do with Anna? Prana is pure consciousness. It is the vital energy that brings everything into being. It lives in the organs of the body and unites all the body into a unit. It is the glue that holds a self-together. Prana is the vital force of energy that controls and governs the universe. Everything in the universe exists because of the movement of energy prana is the force that moves energy.

It is called, ki, chi, vital force or simply energy. It is the movement that defines breath but it is not breath. For anything to exist there must be motion or movement. The light of the universe is movement through space. The entire universe is created through the movement of particles and waves of energy that make up the atoms or the basic structure of all things. That is the true nature of prana it is simply movement. Prana actually means, before breath. It can take on any quality without losing its purity.

Prana gives vital energy to our bodies and gives us the power to think. It can give force to meditation, to sex, to healing, and to love. It is the movement of thoughts in the mind that give birth to the creations found in the physical world. Prana is the pure energy of consciousness.

Yoga teaches that there are five kinds of prana in the body: prana, apana, samana, udana and vyana. There is also the cosmic prana that is the source of the five prana that are confined to the body. The two most common prana of the body are prana and apana. Prana is seated in the head and the heart and apana is seated at the base of the spine. Prana and apana form the polarity of breath. Apana is the downward breath (exhale) and prana is the upward breath (inhale). These two forces give us the power to breathe. Apana is the lunar aspect or feminine end of the polarity spectrum and prana is the masculine or solar aspect.

Yoga is one of the Vedic sciences and prana is a branch of yoga. Yoga has six branches, which include Prana-maya-kosha and Anna-maya-kosha. Some branches deal with the body, some with the mind, and some with self-actualization or enlightenment.

Yoga generally means a union with the divine or God. Yoga in its purist sense is this union. Although yoga can be practiced from the physical aspect, (asanas) it is the all-inclusive aspect of yoga that unites the body and the mind. It is through the discipline of uniting all six branches, that we practice yoga in its purest form. Prana-maya-kosha is simply a method leading us to the vital force and the source of all that exist.

Prana-maya-kosha is a holistic approach that is as old as humankind. It revitalizes the complete human organism in body, mind and spirit. This is the source of true healing, working not on the disease but on the vitalization of health.

Prana and the mind move naturally. Rising and falling, appearing and disappearing commonly referred to as thinking. Prana and mind exist together. Prana is the principle of movement, and the mind is the principle of intelligence. All action requires prana as all action requires at some level intelligence. Slowing the breath, the mind slows its thoughts and a state of meditation is achieved. This is the balancing of the energies of the body-mind and when the energy is balanced and still health exists.

We only have one body; however, that body is made up of layers that vibrate at different frequencies. Quantum physics tells us that if we take gross matter and vibrate it by the speed of light it will change form. Water is an example. Everything in the universe takes on the form of, solid, liquid or vapor. Water is liquid and yet if we increase its vibrating rate (apply heat energy) it becomes vapor and likewise if we slow down its vibrating rate it becomes solid ice.

Our bodies are made up of several layers. The most familiar layer is the aura. It is a layer of energy that surrounds our gross physical body and can actually be seen and recorded through Teslian Kirlian photographs.

We are made up of seven bodies or layers of energy including our gross physical body. The first body is the physical self; the second is the etheric or the vital energetic self also known as the aura; the third is the astral or emotional self; the fourth is the mental self; the fifth is the spiritual or intellectual self; the sixth is the cosmic self or sometimes called the pure intelligent self, and the seventh is like the Tao, impossible to name as it is beyond name and form.

The higher frequency layers have an effect on the lower frequency layers until at last they reach the gross physical layer known as our body. These layers or bodies are interdependent and cannot be separated. As long as consciousness exists the bodies are joined.

One way to understand the energy layers is to think about stress or any other emotional response such as anger or anxiety. Stress like all emotions is perceptions that are subjective. To experience an emotion, we first have the pure thought found in the mental energy layer. The thought takes on the energy of emotion, affecting the energy of the aura and then reaches the gross physical body.

In other words, stress is first perceived and then finally we experience the sensation in the physical body. This is also true of the foods we eat. The energy comes from the outside, ending at the gross physical level. Therefore, if we take in healthy vital foods the body ultimately is the end receiver of this vital energy. Therefore, we should always strive to bring clean and healthy foods to the body-mind.

No doubt you have heard the phrase "Cleanliness is next to Godliness". In yoga this is both external and internal cleanliness. In yoga it is believed that to gain lasting benefits from the practice, it is necessary to maintain a high level of bodily cleanliness. Along with daily bathing and grooming one should practice Anna-maya-kosha or the yoga of diet and fasting.

This practice is also known as purification of the body, and is based upon the concept that as long as the body has impurities the pranic force cannot be collected in the astral or emotional body. If the pranic force cannot be accumulated the mind will not be able to find emotional stability, balance, and quietude, and therefore will not be able to vibrate to its highest level of soulful awareness.

There are four substances which if they accumulate in the body are detrimental to body-mind health and soulful enlightenment.

They are:
1. Lactic acid
2. Toxic gas
3. Waste
4. Phlegm and mucus

1. **Lactic acid** is the build up of metabolic waste products in your muscles. This happens when oxygen is lacking in the breakdown of stored sugars, which supply energy for muscle contraction. The muscles contract until such a build up of lactic acid causes the muscles to stop contracting. This causes exhaustion and fatigue. Thus, a person lacks the mental acuity and physical energy to perform body-mind and soulful task.

2. **Toxic gas** or carbon dioxide (waste product), when combined with water produces an acid that is irritating to the body and nervous system. This irritability is detrimental to serenity and quietude.

3. We need sufficient oxygen to keep the mind alert and assist the body in eliminating **waste**. A buildup of waste causes the mind to become agitated and this in turn causes the liver to be over taxed and disrupts the normal flow of bile. Bile is a molecule that aids in lipid (fat) digestion.

4. An excessive amount of **mucus or phlegm** is a medium for bacteria, as well as inhibits the absorption of prana to the astral body (emotional). This in turn causes one to be sluggish and lacking vitality.

Anna–maya–kosha yoga promotes the elimination of waste from the body through the process of conscious choice making of the foods we take into our bodies. This results from awareness of the process of digestion, assimilation and elimination.

Our modern-day lifestyles have drastically affected our natural power of elimination due to three major factors:

1. Over indulgence in process foods lacking sufficient bulk (fiber) and nutrients
2. Lack of exercise due to sedentary work and lifestyles, as well as non-active play
3. Stress

When the elimination of fecal matter becomes extreme, the fecal matter is drawn into the bloodstream. Because of this, the oxidation of the blood stream is not as thorough. This produces a mental lethargy, or moodiness. The blood that flows through and around the intestines is the same blood that flows through your brain. If the bowels become sluggish, the blood becomes impure. When impure blood goes to the brain it tends to dull consciousness. When this happens, one tends to become depressed, anxious, pessimistic, and soulfully unaware.

Although western science looks upon the body as a single vehicle with many physiological organs, including a brain, yoga like Naturopathy looks at the body as a triune having three distinct parts, as well as a consciousness:

1. The physical body
2. The mind
3. The soul

These three bodies are capable of functioning separately and yet as the same time are interrelated. The interrelationship of these three bodies is what takes the individual to higher states of consciousness. It is known as the temple of the soulful self and is composed of five sheaths.

THE TRIUNE BODY	THE FIVE SHEATHS
Physical body	food sheath –anna-maya-kosha
(sharira)	prana sheath- prana-maya-kosha
Astral body	mind sheath – mano-maya-kosha
(sukshma)	intellectual sheath–vijnana-maya-kosha
Casual body	bliss sheath – ananda-maya-kosha

Maya means temporal and kosha means sheath. These two words together mean the temporary sheath used by the bodies as a means of the expression of consciousness.

Yoga philosophy states that a long life is extremely important in the enfoldment of wisdom and soulful insight. To insure this, we need to remember that behind the physical food sheath (anna-maya-kosha), which is the essence of food is the vital sheath called the prana-maya-kosha, which is prana the link between the physical body and the astral body. A healthy and vigorous vital sheath gives powerful consciousness to our emotional or astral world. Therefore, we should remember this yogi saying, "You are what and how you eat."

It is difficult to prove the existence of prana, however there is a significant factor that separates prana and oxygen. We know that breath is life and that it is the oxygen/carbon dioxide cycle that is known as respiration. If oxygen is life rather than the force of breath being life, why is it when a human is dying one can not be kept alive with oxygen? There is something beyond oxygen that keeps one alive.

This something else is the force that gives rise to the breath, known as prana.

Prana and the triune sheaths are important in establishing a healthy body-mind. If one is going to be successful it is important to have a strong body and a steady mind. However, anyone who has experienced true success knows it takes something more than a body-mind to win. Victory is not achieved by sheer physical strength nor mental determination, but from a deeper level of soulful strength. Prana, the force that gives rise to breath helps us to consciously work the breath so as to bring about the greatest amount of vitality and health.

When your breath is irregular your mind will be scattered and your body will lack energy. Prana-maya-kosha yoga is practiced to:

1. Give greater discipline to the physical body
2. Increase ability to concentrate the mind
3. To realize higher states of consciousness
4. Ability to draw upon that inner strength when needed

The attainment of these four disciplines requires control of the breath, which controls the energy of the body-mind.

The triune body is more than a mass of muscles and nerves. There are also astral channels known as nadis, or nerve points that run through the body. These nadis are points, or channels that are unblocked through the process of acupuncture. The needles are inserted between the nerve points, or at the point of the nadis to release blockages that cause imbalances.

These life currents run through the body-mind. According to yoga these channels become blocked with phlegm, lactic acid, toxic gas and lack of oxygen due to poor diets and lifestyles. The function of yoga is to remove the blockages. When the nadis are cleaned, prana flows through and increases physical strength, concentration and awareness. When the nadis are purified through proper yoga techniques such as Anna-maya kosha and asana work, prana stimulates and vitalizes the gross, subtle and super subtle levels of your being, giving consciousness control over your body-mind.

Your consciousness is the energy that defines you. You are what you think, say and do, so yoga teaches us to always make conscious choices regarding the health of our body-mind. Your body-mind is the temple of the soul. As such we are taught that what we honor is what we become. So, if you consciously choose to honor the body-mind through the practice of Prana-maya-kosha and Anna-maya-kosha you elevate yourself to a higher level of consciousness, where you become the creative principle of your life.

As we move through the next few chapters, remember you don't need to change your diet. Anna-maya-kosha yoga will change your diet, as it teaches you how you truly become what and how you eat. Remember this; you reap in life what you sow. If your focus is radiant health than Anna-maya-kosha yoga is a discipline for you.

ANNA-MAYA-KOSHA-YOGA
THE ESSENCE OF FOOD

The practice of Anna-maya-kosha is the principle of the yoga diet, which states that we should soulfully approach the choice of foods we use to nourish our body-mind. From a soulful perspective we learn to choose wisely with a focus towards balanced health. We should seek to establish balanced health in all aspects of our lives and since food is the substance of continual life, it should reflect the state of our being.

The ancient yogis referred to this as the body and mind mirroring each other. The state of the body reflects one's emotional states and one's emotional state is reflected in the health of the body. Therefore, what we eat truly affects our inner life.

The yogis divided the essence of foods into three major categories. One type of food promotes life, vitality, energy, strength, balance, emotional stability, and health. A second type makes us agitated and scattered and brings illness and pain. Ultimately this high level of agitation leads to exhaustion. A third type makes us sluggish, lethargic and apathetic, also leading to illness and exhaustion.

These three categories of food have been compared to the three primary forces of nature, which are called sattva, rajas, and tamas. These are the Sanskrit (ancient Ayurvedic scripture) names for the three forces responsible for the entire web of creation. They have been compared to the principles of light, motion and gravity. These forces are not only physical forces, but are the underlying psychological forces of emotion.

The sattva, the principle of light is physically, mentally and soulfully uplifting and illuminating. The rajas, the principle of motion keeps the body-mind in constant tension and conflict. The tamas, the principle of gravity, is binding causing us to be creatures of habit, becoming attached to sameness and continuity rather than being spontaneous and innovative.

Yoga means to "yoke", which is all-inclusive and no aspect of life is ignored which includes diet. Our diet, according to Anna-maya-kosha, is the yogic path to purity, evolution, serenity and joy. This of course brings balanced health in the body-mind. It therefore matters what you eat, how much you eat, and when you eat.

On the yogic path we are taught to become the observer of our lives. This of course includes becoming the observer of the effect different foods and the quantities of food have on your body-mind.

According to the ancient yogic scripture, The Bhagavad Gita (XXII. 888) there is three personality types and three categories of foods that support each personality type.

1. **The Sattva personality** – the principle of light, seeks evolution, growth and balance. Their minds are focused on action that is creative, life supporting and healthy. Therefore, they choose foods that are savory, living, healthy, and organic.

2. **The Raja's personality** (most westerners) – the principle of motion, constant motion, mental and physical activity tending towards impatience, impulsiveness and kinetic outlets of all

kinds. The raja personality tends towards foods that are harsh and burning, sharp, spicy and salty.

3. **The Tamas personality** - the principle of gravity, the body-mind does not like to act, prefers routine and sameness becoming overly attached. This person prefers foods that are tasteless, unclean, processed, leftover, stale, and overcooked.

These three categories are not cut and dry. We all contain elements of each; however, one seems to predominate over the others.
We all know the:
Raja type, who is extroverted, impulsive, impatient, agitated and over active.
Tamas type, who is slow to move, resistant to new ideas, hard-core traditionalist for whom the best of life exist in the past.
Sattva type, who is creative, innovative, open to new ideas, growing, expanding and evolving.

The secret of the sattva type is that they have natural healthy desires. They are aware of the choices they make, conscious of their existence. Their focus is positive awareness of the dynamic beauty of life. They have the ability to step forward into the mystery of life (uncertainty) with balance and joyous wonder.

The sattva personality observes each and every choice in life and always strives to make the best choice that will bring the greatest good. In doing so the sattva draws to self the positive energy of good karma, which brings health in its train.

The opposite of healthy desires is *Ama* the Sanskrit word for impurities, which means residual deposits in the cells as a result of improper digestion (which we'll discuss in the section on nutrition and digestion). There is also mental ama, which are negative thoughts and moods.

Mental ama arises from:

1. Negative thoughts based in one or more of the four great passions; deceit, greed, anger and pride, which are the root cause of all negative karma

2. Stress – stress is a perception. What is stressful to one person may not be to another, however, family problems, work tension, moving, loss of a loved one, and divorce seems to head the list of top stressors. There is also "eustress" which is positive stress such as a marriage, a baby, a new job, and a new relationship

3. Apathy – mental inertia

4. Unhealthy environment – physical and mental

5. Contact with other people's negative vibrations or energy

6. Violent, crude, negative movies, books and other forms of entertainment.

Fatigue, disease, anxiety, and depression are the result of negative energy that builds up in the body-mind from both a poor diet and negative emotions.

You cannot force your body to make lifestyle changes. Applying force creates resistance and resistance will chase you all over the place. If you are eating the wrong foods, somewhere in your consciousness there exist a block. To release the block means to become aware, and in the peace and quietude of your inner soulful self to make the conscious choice to change.

If you begin and continue to practice Anna-maya-kosha yoga you will see yourself making healthy choices as you strive to maintain balance and vitality. This is because Anna-maya-kosha is the path of knowledge about the essence of food and our health. Knowledge removes ignorance and when ignorance is removed, we make wiser choices. This means we learn to be in balance with nature, for in nature everything in its natural and healthy course grows and expands. Like the nature of Prana-maya-kosha, the breath of expansion and contraction, Anna-maya-kosha is about finding that perfect rhythm where activity and relaxation support each other.

ALL THINGS IN MODERATION

Anna-maya-kosha yoga promotes radiant health through the conscious focus on the essence of food. Essence means the basic nature, or concentrated substance of something. The purest essence is the highest quality. Many ancient texts are filled with hidden meanings and allegorical stories about the deep and secret mysteries of the transformation of worthless substances into precious essences.

In the days of alchemy (changing form), the alchemist of the Middle Ages sought to transform the baser metals of lead into gold. It was believed that if one could take basic properties, and through a distillation process, remove the impurities the result would be of divine origin. In the alchemist's view, everything from sand and stones, to plants and people had a physical body, a mind, and a soul. The art consisted of dissolving (distillation) the physical body and condensing it into (precious substances), the quintessence of life. This is not unlike the laws of Karma, where we are directed to cleanse and purify over and over until finally, we transcend the birth and death cycles.

Although the mystical works continue to weave the quest for physical mastery into the quest for soulful wisdom, it is the quest for the divine word of God (spirit) that predominated. It was believed that the True Heavenly Stone was in fact the word of God, and that its purpose was to tinge our souls for salvation and eternal life. This divine word would lead one to the universal tincture that in fact, would turn the ordinary into the extraordinary, but could only be found through the word of God.

The work, through its complete understanding of the soul, which was believed to be the only path for those seeking truth, emphasized transmutation of the soul rather than the physical world. Man was presented as iron in unconverted will and purpose, and it is this, as well as all the thoughts of desire, that must be transmuted into the divine essence.

When reunion between the creator and creature was accomplished, the soul was freed of vice, and the heart was dedicated to virtue and the love of all. The knowledge of God was believed to be the first duty of every reasonable being.

The basic foundation of all things was seen as the spirit of God, and their spirit alone may explain all things. The highest unity was revealed through diversity, and the diversity then must return itself to unity.

This unity is the balance of all things. Balance in yoga means to seek balance in all things and in all things to find balance. It is not about aiming for self-denial, but rather the extinction of physical, mental and soulful imbalances. This means that all things should be approached with moderation, which includes diet.

When you realize the inner temple of your own body, you understand the totality of the universe. This simply means that through balance and moderation we reach an understanding of the unification of the opposing forces of the universe; matter and spirit. These two forces bring about an interaction of self-conscious awareness, which produces illumination.

Diet is a very important part of the yoga path as it can bring purity, balance and health to the body-mind. This in turn brings serenity and peace and this leads us to the spiritual path. That is why in yoga we are taught to honor the temple of the soul; the body and the mind. The Hatha Yoga Paadipika recommends a vegetarian diet of ghee, butter, milk, grains, honey, several Indian vegetables and pure water, as well as eating minimally and fasting periodically.

Although most in the West overeat, eat a poor diet, and rarely if ever fast, a traditional ancient yoga diet does not necessarily work in our modern-day culture. When considering a diet, it is important to look at many lifestyle factors. We must take into account that although the ancient scriptures are full of spiritual advice and prescribe a lifestyle of health and balance, evolution, change and different cultures create the need to expand our consciousness and approach to the essence of the foods we eat.

In fact, modern dietician might disagree with all the dairy and fat in the ancient yogic vegetarian diet. Less dairy and fat are usually promoted in a Western healthy diet, as well as, eating less. Very rarely do we see fasting promoted for health.

The ancient scriptures of Anna-maya-kosha yoga are an important source for laying down the foundation of the path of health through the essence of food; however, we should not follow the scriptures blindly. Anna-maya-kosha yoga is a spiritual path, which promotes honoring the body-mind through the essence of food; therefore, we should seek to discover our own optimal diet for our own individual self.

In a world of ever decreasing resources and increasing populations, addressing the issue of food shortages and nutritional content is extremely important. Much of what we eat today is nutritionally void due to over processing and the poor condition of the soil in which our foods are grown.

It is not simply calories that we need to maintain the body-mind, but nutritional whole foods that can be easily assimilated and support the health and balance of the entire body-mind. It's as much about what you eat, as it is about what you don't eat, that counts. This simply means that sometimes it's what you are not eating that is more important to your health than what you are eating.

Good nutrition is not about cure, but about life enrichment. This means that although we need foods to help rebuild and heal the body, the Anna-maya-kosha-yoga approach is a focus of life enhancement and wellness by increasing the life force energies through the choices of foods we eat. If we eat healthy the body-mind finds vitality, strength, and balance and this is what is needed to keep on our soulful path. It has been said that nature provides all that humankind needs to stay healthy and fit. Whole organic natural foods should provide the basis of a healthy diet.

Disciplined eating is considered one of the basic moral observances, or niyamas and one of the basic abstinences, or yamas, which are two of the eight basic stages of the practice of yoga. Yoga teaches us to take care of our body-mind so as to do no harm to both the internal and external environments. Food can uplift, or pollute our being. Only a body that is strong and steady, and a mind that is clear and sharp can serve our soulful awakening. Therefore, Anna-maya-kosha yoga teaches that we should observe what we eat, abstain from harming the body with impure foods and take responsibility for our dietary needs and the health of our body and our mind.

DO NO HARM

Anna-maya-kosha-yoga is the soulful aspect of the essence of food and how our diets affect our entire life force. Food is the essence of life, for without it the body-mind will soon deplete itself of energy. Energy is needed to live a long and fruitful life, which is the path to gaining wisdom and discovering the true purpose of life. The goal, with Anna, is to bridge the distance between balanced health in body-mind and soulful realization.

In astrology an Aspect is the distance between two planets. The distance is measured in degrees and this distance reveals the strength and character of the planetary energy. A trine is a measure of 120 degrees. It is a triangle with three equal sides and is the symbol of good luck.

In Karma yoga (the yoga of one's life work) it is taught that it takes 120 days to change a piece of karma. (Refer to my book – How to Master Karma). Science tells us that it takes approximately 120 days for the red blood cells in the body to change. The cells of our bodies are structures of information directed at keeping the body-mind optimally functioning. Foods (nutrients), oxygen and water are the vital energy and information that are necessary to keep the cells healthy. Therefore, in 120 days we could reprogram the body-mind towards optimal health through dietary changes.

The three-sided trine represents the triad of body-mind-soul, which is our complete self. In yoga it is the realization of all three and then the integration and balance of all three, through the practice of yoga, that brings about optimum in health and balance. This is done through the ritual of eating, as well as exercise such as the asanas.

Since all creatures participate in the ritual of eating, and many eat meat, what does it mean to do no harm?

Ahimsa is the practice of non-violence, and is the foundation of Anna-maya-kosha-yoga; do no harm. However, with humans, when it comes to the practice of non-violence we must take into account class, time, place and circumstances. Class means the station of one's life. For the monk in the monastery the choices of life are far different than the householder. The place in which you live and the times in which you live, as well as the circumstance of your life determine the choices you make. We must first consider circumstance and lifestyles before following a prescribed doctrine, such as, do no harm, to the letter.

 The modern-day world presents us with a different set of challenges than ancient times when the scriptures were written. However, it is clear that the choices we make should be conscious and with the focus on obtaining wisdom.

The intent to refrain from violence and live a harmonious and balanced lifestyle is what should be emphasized. It is conscious choice making as it relates to your own individual enfoldment and awareness that constitutes Anna-maya-kosha-yoga, and not necessarily a vegetarian or vegan diet.

Traditional yogic diet is a lactose vegetarian diet, meaning the inclusion of milk, butter and honey. The Hatha Yoga Pradipika, an ancient yoga manual recommends a variety of grains, honey, milk, ghee, butter, several Indian vegetables and pure water. Eggs are eliminated because they are considered stimulating.

Many modern-day nutritionists would argue that a heavy dairy diet combined with the methods used to produce dairy products does not constitute a health enhancing diet. Most nutritionists support a vegetarian diet, but emphasize the food pyramid as a basis for the structure of a healthy diet.

Research has shown that a vegetarian diet can be healthy if balanced properly. A plant-based diet low in fats and rich in complex carbohydrates has been shown as a preventative for cancer, heart disease, diabetes, gall bladder problems, obesity and numerous other medical conditions. Further a vegetarian based diet frees up grain for human consumption. But is it safe?

THE VEGAN - VEGETARIAN DIET

A variety of whole organic foods from the plant kingdom can provide ample nutrition. The only vitamin not supplied directly from a pure vegetarian diet is vitamin B-12, found almost exclusively in meat.

Complete proteins are necessary for sustaining life. They provide the structure for all living things and participate in the biochemical process enabling living things to perform a wide range of functions. It is impossible not to get enough protein on a well-balanced vegetarian diet. The key word is balance. Getting complete proteins requires the combining of certain foods such as grains and legumes. We'll look at protein requirements and food combining in the section on Conscious Eating.

Anna-maya-kosha-yoga is about the conscious choice of what and how we feed the body-mind. It is done with the intent to do no harm. A conscious lifestyle might include not eating meat, not wearing clothes, or shoes made from animal hides and even to find alternatives to household products and cosmetics that are not tested on animals.

The focus is not so much on vegetarianism as it is on doing no harm by making a conscious choice about what you put into and onto your body. Anna-maya-kosha-yoga teaches that there is an environment within us and outside of us. It is up to each of us to protect and do no harm to that which both belongs to us and belongs to all of us collectively. However, it is not about a dictate, but rather about the freedom to choose what is in the best interest of the individual on a conscious and healthy level.

What may have worked several thousand years ago in a different culture may not work today in our Western culture. The intent should always be to do no harm and to act in such a way that the results are for the greatest good for the majority.

Vegetarianism is much like Anna-maya-kosha-yoga in that when you learn about it, you begin to make subtle changes in the way you look at things. These subtle changes come about with a realization that you are now a little slimmer, a little calmer, a little happier and a little more at peace. Your energy becomes balanced and life is lived in moderation rather than excess.

Vegetarianism and veganism are safe and healthy ways to eat, but not necessary in the practice of Anna-maya-kosha-yoga. Remember we must always be open. Look at the lifestyle and culture of us as individuals, and make choices that are appropriate for us without doing harm to ourselves and to others.

Here we practice the abstention of non-violence. The main source of non-violence or doing no harm is within our minds. It is the mind that manifests harmonious or inharmonious energy. With an unhealthy diet and lifestyle, we are doing harm to our bodies and our minds. The focus should be more on living a healthy lifestyle, rather than whether or not to eat meat.

Before performing any mental or physical action, one should reflect upon the consequences. If the consequences will result in harm to self and/or to others the action should be avoided. The more one develops a sense of non-violence, the more one cultivates a feeling of connection to all things, and therefore will not take any action that will bring harm.

However, self-satisfaction alone cannot determine whether an action is positive or negative. One who feels a sense of satisfaction at the time the action is performed may perform all unrighteous actions such as harming, killing, stealing and lying. The difference between an action that is positive or negative is not whether it gives you immediate gratification, but whether it ultimately results in positive or negative results.

Excess desires lead to greed and greed ultimately leads to disappointment. For as soon as we obtain one thing, we desire ten things and as soon as we obtain ten things, we desire one hundred things. This is the nature of greed and greed leads to violence, which leads to harm.

Non-greed means to recognize your realistic and necessary needs and strive for them. However, you should not reach out beyond your needs. This does not mean we do not have goals, but rather we clearly have defined what we need at each stage of our lives and honestly work to acquire that which will allow us to provide the best without harm.

The soul firmly established in non-harm clearly understand what must be done is this lifetime to bring about a state of balance and health. For from a place of balance the life force energy is gathered together and one moves forward with peace and serenity.

The goal of the practice of non-violence and all the abstinences is to bring about peace of mind. If you are practicing non-harm and do not have peace of mind you will suffer. Taking a vow to practice conscious action without a balanced and peaceful mind might result in a scattered and frustrated being.

If you take a vow to stop eating candy, sugar, meat or coffee but keep thinking about then all day, and then feel guilty and frustrated, it might be better to have some of these things in moderation, and then allow yourself to stop dwelling on the desire. This way you release yourself from a scattered and distracted mind.

Disciplining the body-mind to practice non-violence and non-greed does not mean we need to experience a sense of deprivation, which is why most self-imposed disciplines fail. Rather it means that we act moderately in all things and consciously choose that which will bring us the greatest good.

Anna—maya-kosha yoga teaches us to approach all things with the conscious effort to bring about balance and health. For when the body-mind is in a state of health and balance the soulful self can unfold. Desires scatter our focus.

When giving up a habit, or a food that is not serving your highest good, you may at first struggle with the desire hour by hour, but one year later the struggle may be only for 5 minutes, here and there, and still later the struggle may disappear altogether.

The purpose of abstaining is to bring about peace of mind and balance to the body-mind. When we practice non-harm through the healthy choices we make, peace health and serenity cannot help but appear.

The purpose of yoga is to balance the scattered energies of the subconscious mind so that the conscious actions we take flow and move in balance and harmony. Thoughtfully we can practice Anna-maya-kosha-yoga, which is not a strict prescribed diet, but rather a conscious approach to the healthy essence of the food we eat.

Remember, you are what and how you eat. So, choose today what you will want tomorrow because what you choose today you will need to live with tomorrow.

THE RITUAL OF EATING

Anthropologists believe that the defining moment in the emergence of human culture was as the result of some kind of ritual. Rituals are a part of every religion and all cultures, and food and feasting are important parts of cultural rites. Rites are usually thought of as solemn and ceremonial. Ritual magic claims that; if you follow a certain course of action with dedication and persistence you will be led back to the roots of your own identity, you will learn the truth about yourself and the universe which you inhabit, and the nature of your existence will be transformed.

"Breaking bread" or the ritual of sharing food is a very important aspect of the bonding between humans. According to the Bible God gave humans the seeds and fruits of the earth for food. The promise land flowed with milk and honey. It was literally a cornucopia over flowing with every kind of healthy and healing foods.

> *...A land of wheat and barley, and vines, and fig trees, and pomegranates; a land of oil olive and honey; a land wherein thou shalt eat bread without scarceness, thou shalt not lack anything in it...*
> ~ Deuteronomy 8:8 ~

Nearly every book of the Bible refers to healthy and healing foods, as well as rules for governing, cultivating, preparing and consuming foods. For example; the Talmud, which is the body of the ancient Jewish civil and religious law, tells how to prepare certain foods and certain foods to avoid.

It is the ritual of planting, growing, harvesting, preparing and eating that is an essential part of the evolutionary process of humankind. The seasons, the celebration of harvest and significant points in history are all celebrated through the ritual of eating.

Winter, spring, summer and autumn reconnect us with the rituals of life because every event in life is rich in purpose and meaning. Rituals connect us to both the big and little dramas of life and the greater cycle of continuation. With each passing season we reunite in character and spirit through the depth and character of celebration and ritual. Even the humblest of rituals fill us with power and sometimes take us to places outside of ourselves. These moments of ecstasy fill us with a sense of connection to all that exist.

All living things share the ritual of eating. Eating is a magical rite in which we share food, as it becomes transformed into life giving energy and health. Therefore, all food should be prepared fresh and with positive energy. We should never eat food that is prepared by an angry or hostile person. We should be conscious of what we are feeding our bodies and always think of food as an act of giving from a place of love.

The ritual of healthy eating begins with will power. We should seek to abstain from harm by acquiring the habit of making deliberate choices to eat healthy, while removing nervousness, agitation, anger, and negative energy. The ritual of eating should be the intent to eat healthy in a calm and giving manner. Chew slowly, taste the food and always be calm and thankful. Poor eating habits, agitation, eating too fast and negative energy can do much to bring harm to the digestive system. Even the healthiest of diets can be destroyed by negative and stressful energy.

Giving thanks in the form of a prayer often precedes the ritual of eating. In the West the offering of thanks is often a bowing of the head with the hands in a prayer position as we give thanks for the food before us. Yoga teaches us to also take the time to give thanks for the life-giving force of the foods we are about to put into our bodies. In Anna-maya-kosha-yoga we use mudras and mantras as a gesture of conscious thought, to do no harm and to give thanks for the nourishment of life. A mudra is a hand gesture or symbolic non-verbal language. Hand gestures occur in every culture on Earth and may even hold the key to the origins of human communication. In the yoga mudras, we use the five fingers of the hands to make certain gestures that act upon the unconsciousness.

There are more nerve endings connect to the brain and spinal column on the tips of the fingers, the tips of the toes, the tip of the nose, the tip of the tongue and the lips than on any other part of the body. We use the fingers, nose, lips and tongue in the process of eating. By bringing the fingers together we are stimulating nerve endings that communicate directly to the brain.

Mudras are rebalancing and regenerative. When you press the tips of the fingers together, they radiate energy back to the spinal column producing a generative and healing effect. This in turn sends neurological messages to the brain. Neurologists call this the "imagistic" process of thought. This is the time between the thought turning into words and the ideas emerging.

The mystical symbolism of the fingers is based upon the energies radiating from the subconscious mind. Symbolically these fingers relate to the psycho-mental energies. They are not dealing with the body, but with the subconscious mind patterns, where we find the essence of will power and gain mastery over all the mind's energies that hold us into bad and destructive patterns and habits.

The blessing mudra uses the index finger and the middle finger. It is also called the shanti mudra. The index finger is the symbol of the ego and the energy controlled by the subconscious mind patterning. Its energies produce expansion. The middle finger is the controlling force of our habits and conditioned energies.

To perform the om shanti mudra, place the middle finger on top of the fingernail of the index finger, making a slight bow between the fingers. This little bow between the fingers means that the personality or self is ruled by destiny and not the dictates of the ego. It symbolized the individuality of self and the power to face our destiny with the conscious will power of choice. We can choose how we experience the destiny of our lives and in such a decision, direct the outcome.

The shanti mudra is the food blessing gesture, whereby you touch the edge of the plate before eating, sending positive vibrations to the food. As you touch the side of the plate you silently chant the mantra, Om, shanti, shanti, shanti, which means peace. It is the vibration of love and laughter and reestablishes a sense of tranquility, serenity, harmony and peace.

The word mantra means to continually think to be free. It means to transcend the thoughts that keep us conditioned to negative patterns, and to free us from the limitations of the mind.
Mantras are either:

1. Sattvic which have the power to bring wisdom and compassion
2. Rajasic to produce children, wealth, and worldly success

3. Tamasic or words of power used in rituals and ceremonies

Om, shanti, shanti, shanti, is a tamasic mantra. Om means peace, the first shanti symbolizes serenity and health to the physical body; the second shanti symbolizes calmness and peace of mind; the third symbolizes soulful joy. Serenity and health to the body-mind brings about a state of calmness. This state of calmness brings clarity and this clarity brings the will power to make healthy choices regarding the foods we eat. This is the yogi way. When we choose wisely to eat healthy and life-giving foods, eat slowly, taste and enjoy our foods, and give thanks in a state of love and compassion, we bring health and balance in body, mind, and spirit.

When practicing Anna-maya-kosha-yoga the day will come when healthy nutrition will be unconsciously practiced. It is the easiest of life's gifts to master and practice. All creatures practice the unconscious ritual of eating to sustain life. When we add the conscious act of enhancing our health, we practice Anna yoga.

Begin today to bless the process of giving the body-mind the life force of health through making mealtime a time of soulful work whereby you give thanks for your blessings, and consciously choose to feed the body-mind that which is healthy and balanced. Remember;

Om, shanti, shanti, shanty,
peace to the mind, health to the body,
and joy to the soul.

OBESITY - THE AMERICAN EPIDEMIC

In 1999 the Surgeon General reported that 60 percent of Americans are over weight. In 2002 the Federal Food and Drug Administration reported that 60 percent of Americans are either overweight or obese. The national adult obesity rate has increased by 26 percent since 2008 with the present (2020) obesity rate at 42.4 percent. This is the first time the obesity rate has passed the 40 percent rate.

There are many theories for this epidemic ranging from genetics to super sized meals, fast foods, eating out and sedentary lifestyles. Experts tell us to cut consumption and increase exercise. Intellectually we all know this is good and sound advise, however when emotions and habits come into play, we have a different story.

If we are so smart and have all this good advice why does the average American's weight keep climbing? We can blame it on our modern-day lifestyles, lack of time, food choices which include fast foods, junk foods, and more eating out as well as lack of exercise, but how does that explain the number of Americans who eat healthy and find the time to exercise, avoid fast foods and junk foods, and maintain a healthy and balanced weight?

It probably comes down to that word we all dread to hear "discipline". Self-control or self-discipline is a conscious act to implement behaviors that produce a desired result. It is a sense of focus and commitment. What keeps us from this commitment is resistance.

In Anna-maya-kosha yoga rather than focus on losing weight, we focus on controlling the fluctuating mind through perseverance and nonattachment. By consciously practicing to choose foods that are healthy and life sustaining we learn to honor the body-mind through determined effort. Eventually this effect gives way to the flow of subconscious energy and we act without thinking. We don't think to eat healthy we simply eat healthy. Discipline is not seen as something that is forced upon you, but as something that is cultivated and arises as a result of intension and commitment to the health of one's self.

To have clarity of intension is to have an understanding and to examine what the practice of Anna-maya-kosha-yoga is all about. Why am I practicing the conscious choice of honoring my body-mind through the foods I eat? Is it about my health, my weight, my longevity, my sexual self, my self-image, my moods, or the overall quality of my life?

While intension is clearly a necessary component of self-discipline, commitment is equally as important. It takes a strong sense of commitment to discipline the self to focus the mind and keep it focused on a desired goal. Most people would like to make commitments, but say they would like to know how things would turn out before making the commitment. However, if you know how things are going to turn out in life, it doesn't take much of an effort to make a commitment! What makes someone commit to Anna-maya-kosha-yoga is not how things will turn out, but rather choosing to practice because one believes it is the best course of action.

When you observe eating healthy and resist the urge to indulge your cravings, you consciously choose to do what will create the highest and greatest good. Consciously choosing to do no harm you express a trust and faith in yourself. This is the practice of nonattachment.

Nonattachment does not mean we need to let go of the material world. It simply means we need to let go of our attachment to things. This means we release ourselves from the cravings and desires. We surrender and let go, but not blindly. It means we acknowledge things the way they are instead of looking at things as the way we think they should be.

Instead of resisting and blaming ourselves for less than perfect choices, we simply learn to clarify our intentions and make the commitment to accept where we are at, detach from guilt and use our will power to choose, that which serves the highest good.

Self-discipline teaches us that nothing in life comes instantaneously. Life is a long learning process. No path through life is without difficulty, so rather than trying to avoid difficulty we experience the freedom to choose the challenge of change and growth. Freedom is never found through resistance, but rather through the process of choice.

The question is simply this; would I rather face the difficulties of a challenge or remain resistant to conscious choice and live without the positive effects of practicing Anna-maya-kosha-yoga?

Another aspect of obesity is eating disorders. Binge eating is often connected with obesity. Bulimia and anorexia nervosa are eating disorders often associated with very thin people. All three are grounded in a ritual of maladaptive behavior that brings a familiar, though painful and paradoxically comfort to those who use the rituals of starvation, binging, or purging in order to cope.

Binge eating with or without purging, extreme fasting, excess exercise and rigid food restrictions are signs of eating disorders. Individuals report an almost meditative quality in the repetitive mindless quality of their eating. It is a ritual of control in a world that seems out of control.

Most people with eating disorders are seriously cut off from their feelings and body sensations. They often will report that they have no realistic sensation of their body. There is both the denial of the largeness of the body and a failure to see the thinness of the body. Stress, depression and anxiety rule, as feelings of self-hatred are focused on the body. Whether over weight, emaciated, or of normal weight, a person with an eating disorder will see their body as an obstacle to getting what they want out of life. The focus becomes an obsession with the parts of the body the person hates.

Anna-maya-kosha-yoga teaches that the body is more than simply an object to be judged by its outward appearance. The body is an extension of the mind and as such can give us sensual pleasure. Anna-maya-kosha yoga teaches us to reach a place of quietude and in this quietude, we can introduce positive messages. This is more than simply introducing affirmations. It is about tapping into the subconscious energy of self and learning to let go of the negativity and competitiveness that is inherent in our Western world.

Anna-maya-kosha-yoga removes the guilt and the judgment and introduces us to a world of empowerment, direction and choice. The obsessive nature of eating disorders imprisons us in a web of fears and doubts. Anna-maya-kosha-yoga teaches us to let go and shift our focus from resistant control to a focus on health and balance. In that split second between thought and action, we breathe and then act in the way that produces the greatest good for us. When we are anchored in our balanced nature, we see things as they really are; simply the processes of growth and change presented by life to bring about wisdom. Grounded we move with grace and ease and learn to choose with the concept of do no harm.

Anna-maya-kosha-yoga encourages us to inspect how and what we eat. It emphasizes self-love by feeding the body-mind with life sustaining and life enhancing nutrients. Like all the other branches of yoga, Anna-maya-kosha-yoga supports non-competition, non-judgments, self-love, and balanced health. By practicing conscious eating, we have the potential to free ourselves from the ravages of obesity, over weight, and eating disorders.

Anna-maya-kosha-yoga reminds us to use food and diet to become aware of how the body-mind feels and reacts. Honor self through good nutrition, which is the fundamental principle of promoting the ideals of a healthy life. Anna-maya-kosha-yoga means to eat consciously, for truly you are what you eat!

BALANCE IN ALL THINGS

Anna-maya-kosha yoga is not aimed at self-denial, but rather the removal of negative though patterns that keep us caught up in the web of destructive behavior. This destructive behavior produces imbalances in the body-mind. Bringing the body-mind into a state of balance we achieve a state of health found in the perfect balance and rhythm of nature. When all of your energy is in perfect rhythm and balance there is no room for disease. Anna-maya-kosha yoga teaches us to seek balance in all things and in all things to find balance. This is achieved through an understanding of moderation in all things.

Moderation is found through abstaining from greed and gluttony. It is the balancing of the opposing forces of the universe. In moderation we never over extend ourselves nor over indulge. We lift ourselves from the intellectual and into the full experience of life.

The experience of modern-day life certainly can take us beyond moderation and into excess. Last year Burger King spent $287 million promoting its products while the US Government spends about $900 million promoting good nutrition. You would think this would be helpful and yet Sugar consumption has reached an all time high of an average of 152 pounds a year per person.

In 1979 food consumption outside the home was 37% of the average Americans budget; in the 1990s, 47% of the budget was spent on food outside the home. On average we now spend about 60% of our food budget on snacks and foods outside the home.

In 1970, Americans spent about $6 billion on fast food; today the average is more than$110 billion. "Americans now spend more money on fast food than on higher education, personal computers, computer software, or new cars. They spend more on fast food than movies, books, magazines, newspapers, videos, and recorded music-combined." – Fast Food Nation: The dark Side of the All-American Meal.

Ordering a super sized meal at MacDonald's is the equivalent of getting 1500 calories in one meal! This is the total number of calories a semi-sedentary middle-aged person should be getting each day. With all the eating out and grabbing fast food on the run, is it any wonder that Americans are getting fatter!

Moderation requires a sense of self-discipline. Anna-maya-kosha-yoga, remember is not about self-denial, but rather about the conscious choices we make to insure balance and health to the body-mind. There is a big difference between denial and support. It is simply a matter of perspective. The behavior of choosing healthy foods over fast foods is the same, but the attitude and perspective is what makes all the difference in how we experience our choices. When the experience becomes one of honoring and loving, the denial gives way to balance and harmony.

THE SCIENCE OF EATING

E ating is a complex behavior that depends upon an array of social, physiological and mental influences. Regulating our food in-take is complex. Besides needing a balanced diet, we also need different amounts of nutrients to help us digest and assimilate our food. For example, the more carbohydrates we eat the more thiamine- B1- we need. B1 acts as a catalyst to effectively use carbohydrates as fuel. B1 is found in organ meats such as liver, brown rice, rice bran, egg yolks, soybeans, poultry and fish.

Digestion begins in the mouth as food is chewed and mixed with saliva, which contains enzymes that break down carbohydrates. This is why it is important to chew slowly. When swallowed food travels to the stomach where it mixes with hydrochloric acid and several enzymes the food is digested. From the stomach the food passes to the small intestine, which contains enzymes that help digest the protein, fats and carbohydrates. From the small intestine digested materials are carried throughout the blood stream. If more carbohydrates, proteins and fats are absorbed than used, the excess is stored as fat. The body converts nutrients to glucose, which is the body's primary fuel.

Glucose is by far the most important fuel used by the brain. The brain never sleeps and over all uses about 20 percent of the body's energy. It requires constant oxygen, which it receives from the bloodstream. It uses approximately 25 percent of all oxygen inhaled. Therefore, proper oxygen intake is essential for optimum brain functioning.

The heart, liver, fat cells, muscles, and lungs all compete with the brain for glucose. So, in order to get enough glucose to the brain you must maintain a proper diet. To function properly the daily requirements of the brain are four ounces of glucose, as well as potassium, sodium, unsaturated fatty acids, amino acids (proteins), vitamins, minerals and about 400 calories. Researches suggest a diet of fruits, vegetables, whole grains, rice bran, nuts, soybeans, fish, kelp, salmon, sardines and poultry to improve brain functioning.

It was proposed in 1953 by Jean Mayre that glucose to the cells is the primary base of hunger and satiety. However, in 1977 a study was conducted, (Strickland, Rowland, Saller & Freidman) using fructose which cannot be converted to glucose but was also shown to suppress hunger. The conclusion is that hunger and satiety are not based upon glucose levels alone, but on a variety of nutrients.

The level of glucose in the blood varies little under normal conditions. Even under periods of prolonged fasting the livers converts' stored glycogen, fat and proteins into glucose to maintain blood glucose levels. However, availability of glucose to the cells can vary based upon the blood levels of two pancreatic hormones, insulin and glycogen.

Insulin facilitates the entry of glucose into the cells, which may use the glucose for current energy needs, or stores it as glycogen. Glycogen, a hormone released by the pancreas stimulates the liver to convert glycogen to glucose thus raising blood glucose levels. After meal insulin levels rise, glucose enters the cells and hunger decreases. As time passes blood glucose levels drop, the pancreas starts releasing more glycogen and less insulin, and hunger returns.

Generally, when insulin levels are high, hunger is low. However, if insulin levels remain high and glycogen levels remain low well after the last meal, the body continues to move glucose into the cells, and the liver cells and the fat cells continue to store it as the glycogen and fat. Obese people produce more insulin than do people of normal weight. This is because people produce more insulin when they eat and when they are getting ready to eat. If you eat more and more often you are producing excess insulin (Johnson and Wildman, 1983). Their high levels of insulin cause more of their food to be stored as fat and therefore appetite returns sooner. It becomes a viscous cycle.

METABOLIC RATE

M ost of the calories people consume are not used for exercise, but for basal metabolism; the energy that is used to regulate body temperature and other constant activities. Studies have shown that people vary in their basal metabolic rate although they do not vary much in terms of their body temperature.

People with higher metabolic rates produce more heat than others, but do not radiate it to their environment. People with lower metabolic rates generate less heat but conserve it better.

Because of the difference in metabolic rate one person will lose weight while eating what appears to be a large amount, and another will gain weight while eating a moderate amount. Metabolic rates vary depending upon a variety of factors, probably including genetics. However, genetics also influences the structure and type of body, meaning a heavy framed person is genetically predisposed to a larger frame, but not necessarily a slower metabolism. Although there appears to be a relationship between weight and genetics, there has not to date been a longitudinal study to draw conclusions.

In fact, researchers in a study reported in the Journal of Obesity found that although metabolism does seem to slow slightly after 30 it is lifestyle factors such as eating habits and lack of exercise that cause weight gain and not metabolism. Further the study found that women who agreed with the statement "Some are born to be fat, others thin;

there is nothing I can do" had a higher body-mass index than those who disagreed. Therefore, while body shape is fated, weight is not.

What researchers do believe is that by lowering caloric intake the metabolic rate decrease. And because you burn fewer calories people who yo-yo diet, gain, lose, gain and lose often find that it becomes more difficult to lose on each succeeding diet.

Regardless of how much you weigh, metabolism is likely to slow at midlife largely due to the fact that we begin to lose muscle tone. This is known as Sarcopenia which means age related decline in lean mass muscle. After about age 45 aging starts to accelerate. Your weight may stay the same, but the lean muscle slowly begins to erode. Yo-yo dieting can make Sarcopenia worse because dieting depletes lean muscle. Because lean muscle uses more calories than fat, when you diet you reduce the body's ability to burn fat and your metabolic rate drops.

The only way to reverse and stop Sarcopenia is to exercise consistently. Weight training boost lean muscle mass, reduces fat and therefore burns more calories and speeds up your metabolism. A low-fat moderate diet of fruits, vegetables, complex carbohydrates and protein along with regular weight bearing exercise will reverse Sarcopenia. Weight bearing exercise should be done at least three times per week for 30-45 minutes.

Be patient and be consistent. Consistent self-discipline is the master key to achieving your goals.

Several phytonutrients have been found to be important to overall health and for the metabolic process. Coenzyme Q10 is a vitamin like substance resembling Vitamin E but may be a more potent antioxidant. Phytonutrients are vitamin like substances acting as antioxidants. As we age our body's natural ability to produce Q10 declines.

Lipoic acid is another phytonutrient. It is an important compound for producing energy in the muscles and is an important part of the antioxidant system.

This important nutrient unlocks the energy from food, directing calories into energy production and away from fat production. Lipoic acid also stabilizes blood sugar levels and reduces glycation; the damage done to the body by excessive sugar. Glycation often leads to diabetes, heart disease and accelerated aging.

Lipoic Acid is referred to as a "conditionally" essential antioxidant nutrient. This means that although we produce some lipoic acid in our bodies, for optimum health we must obtain it from the foods we eat. This single nutrient, Lipoic Acid, has amazing importance to our body, best described by its nickname" the metabolic antioxidant". Lipoic acid is a coenzyme that is involved in metabolism (energy production) and is a universal antioxidant that directly and indirectly helps to protect our bodies from stress.

However, like Q10 our body's ability to produce Lipoic Acid declines as we age. So, what does this all mean to a weight management program? These nutrients can help our body metabolize more efficiently. Especially as we age, we need to supplement our diets with Q10 and Lipoic Acid.

Q10 can be found in sardines, spinach, peanuts and beef heart. Lipoic Acid as well as Q10 can be found in stabilized rice bran.

Now you can see how complex carbohydrates, proteins and fats, from the right foods in the right portions will help us to achieve success in the weight management program.

There is a saying about success. Success is precision. But what is precision? It's the right amount of energy, aimed in the right direction, with the right amount of force, at the right time. Successfully managing your weight is nothing more than being focused precisely on your health.

Basically, the low carbohydrate and high protein diet is based upon the insulin resistance theory. However, there is a draw back to excessive protein in the diet. Although it is good to cut out simple carbohydrates, we know that we need to get complex carbohydrates to help the body metabolize efficiently. Again, our moods and attitudes have as much to do with weight loss and management as our daily intake of calories and exercise.

Let's look at the diet myth.

THE DIET MYTH

A myth is a tradition that cannot be verified by fact, although it often happens that a myth turns out to be grounded in fact. A myth is a story serving to explain some phenomena. In this case it is the myth about diets. Simply cut calories and give up "bad" foods forever and you will be thin and svelte. If only it were that easy! Some people are born thin and never have to worry about weight gain! Not true!

Americans spend approximately upwards of $60 billion on weight loss programs, pills and foods. Even with that kind of spending, the weight loss industry experiences a 95% failure rate. According to the International Journal of Obesity, the failures are due to a feeling of deprivation.

It is estimated that two-thirds of the American population is over weight with obesity being a major risk factor in diabetes, heart disease and death. Obesity is defined as being overweight by 20 percent of desired weight and can reduce life span by 10 years, not to mention its negative effects on the quality of our lives.

Over the last century numerous extreme diets have been promoted. Recently the market placed has seen an avalanche of diet programs, each proclaiming to be the answer to the ever-present search for a weight loss program that both works and keeps the weight off. Most of these diets are really diet fads from the 1970's that are making resurgence. For example, the high protein, low carbohydrate diet is really the old "Scarsdale Diet."

Thankfully there are many Doctors and Nutritionist who are attacking these diet plans and trying to establish dietary guideline that work.

Regarding the high protein diet, a lack of fiber in the diet can cause constipation, which leaves toxins in the body and can weaken it. Too much acid in the body, which is the result of excess proteins, can cause damage to the kidneys. And once you stop the diet and go back to your old routine, the weight comes back.

Excess weight also causes bone and joint problems, in addition to sleep and breathing problems, high cholesterol, gout and gallbladder problems. Blood sugar imbalances are also seen in over weight adults. The New England Journal of Medicine reported that researchers over a 32-year period followed about 300 people in the famous Farmington health Study.

The study found that those who used one fad diet after another to lose 15-30 pounds continually put the pounds back on and they reported that people who continually lose and gain weight appear to have a higher risk of health problems.

Most experts warn that dieters usually put the weight back on over a two-year period. It all seems very discouraging!

Although Doctors have been mostly focused on the physical health risk of obesity, they are now starting to pay attention to the psychological factors. In fact, the psychological aspect may be the most adverse effect of obesity.

Further the psychological (mind) connection with the physical (body) self does in fact determine a great deal of our health. The mind-body connection is a major factor in determining the quality of our lives. Our physical relationship with food has a direct connection with our psychological connection with control.

What is control? It is grounded in our attitudes and beliefs and as any good student of persuasion knows, the most difficult thing to change in an individual is their beliefs and attitudes.

If we don't get quick results, we get frustrated and give up, or we may lose the weight and then go back to our old ways and regain. This is called "yo-yo" dieting and is very detrimental to your health.

What is needed is the right attitude to lose the weight and then the right attitude to keep it off. It is about changing your lifestyle and deciding to live a healthy life. This of course is not an easy task. Takes work - that's karma.

Most of our individual differences such as heredity, gender, social class and ethnicity are factors over which we have little or no control. What we can control is our own personal habits. Health habits will play a major role in how you experience the physical and mental changes of aging, the degree of good health you will have and the longevity of your life.

Perhaps it comes as no surprise that young people have unhealthy lifestyles. They tend to skip breakfast, snack on junk food, drink to excess and smoke. The US National Center for Health Static's, show that low health habits usually improve with age, with exception for obesity and getting too little sleep.

Of course, one of the reasons that we disregard our health in our youth is that we have difficulty in seeing and accepting that we will age and that our current behavior will have a direct link to the long-term outcomes of our health and our lives. We tend to be more optimistic about our own being, assuming we won't get sick or get addicted to a substance. We also tend to make decision based upon immediate reward.

Public health information about the merits of a healthy diet and exercise has helped to make us better informed. That does not mean however that we make better choices.

What we do know is that middle age folks are more likely to adhere to better health practices than the young and that women tend to follow better health practices than men. They are also more likely to get regular check ups and see a dentist.

Another characteristic having a direct bearing on health is personality. From a study done by Paul Costa and Robert McCrae (1980), a dimension called neuroticism or the mental disorder of anxieties, compulsions, obsessions and phobias have a link to smoking, drugs, alcohol and other addictive behavior patterns.

Another study conducted by David McClelland (1989) showed a link between a man's high-level need for power and drinking problems. They are more susceptible to disease because their lifestyle leads them into more stress, which in turn suppresses the immune system.

A sense of control seems to be the deciding factor in one's health. Those who believe they have control over their lives believe that they have the ability to perform some action, behavior, or have control over the environment that will give them control over their lives.

It seems that there is a direct link between personality and health and thus our personality influences our health habits, such as eating a sensible diet. Further it appears that a sense of control and optimism is an important personality characteristic when it comes to changing and implementing healthy lifestyle standards. With control we make better choices.

The myth about diets is not grounded in fact, but rather a story to keeps us spending money and failing, when the real fact is that those who believe they have control over their lives do in fact control their lives; body, mind and soul.

THE THREE LIFE STYLE CHANGES THAT WORK!

No matter what anyone tells you there are really only three things that will bring about a life of health and balance. Are you ready? It's no great revelation that:

Eating natural, in proportion and sensibly - **choice**
Exercising every day - **discipline**
A positive mental attitude - **faith**

These are the three keys to success, whether it is weight loss, or any other element of your life. Sensible, right? Then why is it so difficult? Sensibility to most of us seems boring. It lacks the passion and excitement of pushing the envelope, of tasting the richness of life. It smacks of responsibility and balance.

Natural for many of us is so far removed from our lifestyles that we have forgotten what things really taste like, smell like and feel like. Our taste buds and sense of smell have been corrupted by a synthetic world.

Proportion means only enough to satisfy a need. In our society we always want more. We no longer eat or consume to live, but consume on all levels to satisfy our want to have more! Bigger, faster and more is supposed to bring us happiness and fulfillment. Sadly, this mass consumption results from a lack of control and a lack of contentment and does not bring us happiness.

Although we all know we should eat healthy and do some form of exercise each day, it is easy to make exercise and healthy food choices low on the priority list. After all it takes time and effort, and we have so many other important things to do.

Probably the most difficult thing to change is our attitudes. Attitudes are framed around beliefs and become an intrinsic part of our personality.

Why do we develop positive or negative attitudes? The answer lies in the motivational factors within us that bring us satisfaction. Satisfaction is not necessarily a positive thing. Whatever the original motivational drive, the behavior associated with this drive becomes fixed and enlarged over time. In other words, if the original motivation was to satisfy a state of loneliness and boredom by eating, over time this drive becomes fixed and enlarged within our personality.

One of the prevailing drives for humans is to be internally consistent, meaning to have balance and harmony in our lives. However, researchers seem to agree that individuals are not fully aware of their attitudes, and this may account for the inconsistencies. Unless a situation brings the internal conflict to the surface the inconsistencies may go unnoticed.

If we are forced to recognize inconsistencies in our attitudes, we become uncomfortable and seek to resolve the conflict through attitudinal adjustment.

Although our attitudes may greatly change, our basic values change very little over a lifetime. We defend our values through selective perception. We see, hear and assimilate only what supports our way of thinking and disregard whatever challenges our beliefs.

Attitudes have three essential characteristics or dimensions; direction (positive, neutral or negative), intensity (strength with which they are held) and saliency (the perceived importance to the individual). If we want to change an attitude, we first need to look at the dimensions. If an attitude such as anger is strong and intensely held, it will be difficult without a crisis of sorts to change.

We all have a set of feeling and thoughts about ourselves that are acquired from the views of other people. That is why our experiences influence our attitudes.

So, if our attitudes are ingrained, how can we change a negative attitude into a positive attitude? First, we need to become aware of the fact that we all seek out information that is consistent with our held attitudes.

To change an attitude, we need to look at the relationship of new information to the attitudes currently held, the way in which the information source is perceived and the nature of the new information itself.

Let's say your attitude is that you just can't seem to keep your weight under control. A new source of information comes in and says you can do it with a little adjustment to your lifestyle. If the information, the source and the relationship to your currently held attitude is accepted, you will be open to making the changes.

So, the very first thing you need to do is develop a positive attitude that doesn't say "I can't" but only says "I will try." Attitudes are simply imposed points of view. They are simply energy that has taken form in the way you act and conduct your life. The energy can be rearranged and with it will come a different form to your life.

It is not the physical world that imposes limitation on us, but the world of thoughts and feeling, which are our attitudes. You can create whatever image you desire simply by changing your thoughts. But it is important to remember that energy like every thing else in nature takes time to organize and grow. So, it takes focus and determination to change.

What motivates us to make an attitudinal adjustment? Theorists tell us that it takes a crisis of sorts. However, with or without a crisis it is simply the ability to adopt a posture of self- love instead of self-hate. Once we develop a state of self-love, we begin to see the potential within. It is the realization that we have given the substance (food, cigarettes, drugs, alcohol, sex, spending, gambling, etc.) more power and control over our lives than we have.

The material substances of the world now dictate the nature of our being and the nature of our health on all levels, body, mind and soul. We have given away the freedom of choice and become enslaved to the substance.

With this we become addicted to drama, stress, anxiety, depression and fear. We become addicted to negative attitudes. This negativity then makes it impossible to find our way back to the true nature of our being which is a state of health, balance, harmony and happiness. To find balance, harmony and happiness is the reason for our existence on earth. We just need to find our way back onto the path.

To change our lifestyles, we need to change our attitudes toward others, the world, and ourselves. Learning to love and honor ourselves we take the first step towards implementing a lifestyle of health and with this comes first an acceptance of the uniqueness of each of us and on a deeper level the unity of all.

The first law of thermodynamics tells us that energy is never lost it simply changes form. Since you are nothing more than an energy field, nothing that you do is ever lost, but simply manifest into another form. To change your form (health) simply change the method of energy you use. It is simply a matter of balancing, integrating and harmonizing the energy of the body, the mind, and the soul.

HIGH PROTEIN DIET

The basis of the high protein diet is the elimination of carbohydrates. It is further based upon the insulin resistance aspect and the metabolism of fat.

According to a survey conducted in 1983 by the National Center for Health statistics the number one food consumed by most Americans is white bread, rolls and crackers, or purely simple carbohydrates. Number two is donuts, cookies and cakes or simple carbohydrates and fat. The number three position is held by alcoholic beverages which are really sugar. These numbers are still true today.

Sugar the Protein Diet claims is what is making American's fat. If they would simply give up their addictions to carbohydrates, they would lose weight and maintain their weight. Dietary fat they go on to say only causes problems when combined with carbohydrates. Further, that fat is the material that makes cholesterol and that although it is true that if you eat a lot of fat your cholesterol levels will rise, it's all dependent upon eating carbohydrates at the same time. If you reduce the level of insulin, the cells won't convert fat to cholesterol.

The conclusion is that if you eat excess carbohydrates and low protein you will gain weight and always have a weight problem. Excess is the key word. If you eat an excess of anything toxicity will ensue.

Although it is true that controlling your carbohydrate intake is both beneficial to your weight management and to your health, it is difficult to fully support a diet that allows you to eat excess protein, fats and preservatives. These diets allow you to eat fats, processed foods and foods such as sausages that are full of preservatives and artificial flavorings.

Most of these diet plans are based around a reward system of allowing you to have certain foods if you have been "good" all day and stick to the diet. Again, we find reinforcement with food. You get a "bad" food reward for being good.

One so called reward meals diet says you can eat carbohydrate rich foods only one meal a day, eat as much as you want, but do it in 60 minutes! After the 60 minutes, no more eating! I bet in sixty minutes a lot of so called "reward" food can be consumed!

The writers probably meant that in your reward meal you can eat a variety of foods and believe that you will act responsibly and make good choices. But isn't that the problem, we've been making the wrong choices?

According to dietary standards we need to eat a well-rounded group of foods, which include, complex carbohydrate, proteins and fats. Balance and proportion are the key. The human body only needs so much to operate at efficiency. More is not better.

These diets say that our daily requirements for protein are determined by the amount of lean body mass and the level of activity. If we are a moderately active person (exercise 20 minutes 3 times per week) you would require about 60 grams of protein. That's about 20 grams per meal.

The American Diet Association's dietary guideline says that 48 percent of our daily intake should be complex carbohydrates and 12 percent should be proteins. However, when it comes to carbohydrates the key is complex. This is what the body uses for energy. However, if the diet is deficient in carbohydrates (as in a high protein, high fat diet) the body uses the protein for energy. Normally protein is used to build and repair the body. If we use it for energy, how can we build and repair?

Because carbohydrates are the source of glycogen, the most efficient fuel for aerobic exercise, getting adequate amounts of complex carbohydrates while implementing an exercise program to both lose and maintain weight seems vitally important.

Most Americans eat in excess of the amount of protein needed. The Recommended Daily Allowance is based upon the ideal weigh of the individuals. The average adult requires about 0.36 grams of protein per pound of body weight. For the average 125 lb. woman that would be 45 grams per day.

Excess protein like calories from any other source are stored as fat. Too much protein whether ingested through foods or supplements produces excess nitrogen (acid) in the body and the kidneys and liver must work harder to eliminate this excess. The kidneys also require more water to dilute the nitrogen for elimination; this water requirement may lead to hydration.

Although it seems that we eat far too much simple carbohydrates in our modern-day diets, we do need adequate protein to support growth. Life remember is about balance and moderation.

Food provides us with two things, energy and the raw material needed to build and sustain life. There are six classes of food that we need, carbohydrates, proteins, fats, vitamins, minerals and water.

Your body does not obtain energy from vitamins, minerals and water. Vitamins are organic molecules that perform functions such as helping the body form red blood cells and "unlock" the energy in carbohydrates, proteins and fats.

Although required in small amounts each of the 13 different vitamins plays a vital role in your body's ability to function. For example, riboflavin and niacin, two of the B vitamins are used to make coenzymes that are used in cellar respiration.

Minerals are inorganic substances that move through the body as ions dissolved in blood and other fluids. Calcium for example we all know helps to build strong bones. Magnesium assists in the release of energy from carbohydrates, fats and proteins.

Water provides the medium in which all of the body's functions take place. The atoms that make up the water molecules are also held within the bonds of the energy molecules.

When you eat foods that are full of preservatives and additives you are putting toxic chemicals into your body. So, the body has to work hard to remove these. This taxes our energy making it difficult for the body to do its work.

The high protein diets tell us we can eat plenty of cheese, nitrates and Nutra Sweet. Although cheese in limited qualities is not going to hurt you, it is high in fat. What's more some are also high in the heavy metal aluminum.

Aluminum, which is a heavy metal, does cause poisoning in the body. Symptoms ranging from forgetfulness, headaches, gastrointestinal disturbances, weak aching muscles and symptoms similar to Alzheimer's disease have been reported. Aluminum is found in deodorants, white flours, breads, water, baking powder, in processed foods such as pickles, beer, parmesan cheese and American cheese. The food products having perhaps the highest aluminum content is a cheeseburger. This mineral is added to the cheese to assist it in melting over the burger.

The point is that if we really want to eat healthy (and that should be the main emphasis) we need to eat natural. The more natural we eat the better our selection. If we can eat free of pesticides and poisons, we will not only ensure better health, but will also be able to control our weight.

Many of the health-related problems facing us today, including obesity have direct correlation to not only the quantity of food that we eat, but also the quality.

THE DIGESTIVE PROCESS
~ WHAT ABOUT FIBER?

The process of digestion is how we obtain the nutrient and energy from the foods that we eat. Food particles are broken down into small molecules that are absorbed by the body.

Chemically digestion is carried out in three ways:
1. By Hydrochloric acid which denatures the protein particles
2. By bile salts that separate the large lipids into smaller lipids
3. By highly specified enzymes that help cleave (split) certain chemicals

During digestion proteins are unfolded by hydrochloric acid and then split into peptides and individual amino acids by protease enzymes. Starch and glycogen are digested to sugars by amylase. Triglycerides are digested to fatty acids and glycerol by lipase.

The digestion of foods yields no usable energy, but rather changes the diverse array of molecules into simple molecules that can be used by the cells for cellular respiration. During cellular respiration ATP molecules are produces providing energy for the body.

Any intake of food in excess of that required to maintain the blood sugar level and the glycogen reserves in the liver results in two situations. Either the excess glucose is metabolized by the muscles and other cells of the body, or it is converted to fat. Only when the energy needed to run the body (move muscles and digest foods) is supplied will the excess be stored as fat.

Proteins, lipids and carbohydrates provide more than just energy. They also provide the raw material to build and sustain the body. In fact, proteins are what we use to build the body. Proteins contain amino acids, which are necessary for building and maintaining the body. Unfortunately, many of the proteins that contain these amino acids are high in fat and cholesterol. A high percentage of fat in the diet has been shown to be related to heart disease and obesity.

If we take away the complex carbohydrates that give us energy and then rely solely upon our proteins, eventually there is bound to be a malfunction. Excess proteins cause excess acid in the system.

As we age our digestion systems due to wear and tear, poor eating habits, and heavy metals and toxins from the foods we eat, tend to slow down. This makes it more difficult to get the appropriate nutrients. Our body produces less hydrochloric acid, which aids in the digestive process. One of the ways to combat this is to get more potassium in the diet. Apple cider vinegar has been shown to assist the digestive system in providing hydrochloric acid. Apple cider vinegar is high in potassium. Take a tablespoon in a glass of water two to three times per day. You can add honey but remember honey adds calories.

We get fiber from complex carbohydrates. Fiber in necessary for proper digestion and elimination of toxins from the body. Recently the American Cancer Association has declared that fiber in the diet is not necessarily a deterrent to colon cancer. However, they did not say to eliminate fiber. It is an important part of the digestive process and complex fibers contains many nutrients that are needed by the body.

Studies have shown however, that dietary fiber reduces cholesterol and therefore is a preventive substance regarding heart disease.

There are seven forms of fiber, cellulose, lignin, gums, mucilage's, pectin, hemicellulose and bran. All of these fibers are found in the natural foods that we eat. The problem is that through the processing and milling process much of our modern-day diet is void of fiber.

Rice Bran has been considered to be of the most wasted foods on our planet. Modern technology now allows us to preserve these important nutrients. The key is to stabilize the rice bran in its natural state. To make brown rice, manufacturers remove the outer layer of the rice bran. Within a very short time this outer layer, which contains important nutrients and antioxidants, goes rancid due to its unstable state. Technology now has the ability to stabilize this outer layer.

Stabilized rice bran is one of the most powerful forms of phytochemicals or plant compounds of any food known to humankind. So not only is it an excellent fiber, but it also supplies vitamins, minerals and other nutrients including essential amino acids, needed to promote health.

Constipation combined with digestive problems is the underlying cause of nearly every ailment. So, we need fiber to help the body eliminate toxins. Again, stabilized rice bran is an excellent fiber and will promote elimination.

A correct, balanced and healthy diet should have fiber in it. It is also important to get plenty of exercise, which we'll discuss later.

Keep in mind that nothing in the universe stays at peak performance at all times. Times of stress and excess strain on the body increases our daily needs. Every one and everything experiences cycles- we all have highs and lows, calm and chaos. We must constantly work to maintain healthy levels of being. By adhering to a well-balanced program of exercise, rest, play and good nutrition we are giving ourselves the best gift of all…a healthy body, mind and soul.

Always add a positive state of mind to any program of healthy living. It is the combination of all aspects of health that work together synergistically to provide optimum health.

There are many factors that lead to disease. However, we know that a healthy, natural and portioned diet combined with exercise, play, rest and a great attitude make for a healthy body, mind and soul.

Basically, we need to eat as natural as possible. When you choose natural foods, you are both getting the nutrients you need and more than likely controlling the caloric intake. Remember it is processed foods that contain many hidden useless calories. Avoid them!

The best diet is one that is natural, being high fiber, low fat, low sugar and moderation in lean and healthy protein. Before we look at how to create a basic diet, let's look at the subject of supplements.

SUPPLEMENTS
~ SHOULD WE?

In an ideal world we would eat a natural diet and get all the nutrients we need. But as we all know this is not an ideal world. Pollutants, eroding soils, quality of foods, stress and every day event can rob us of needed nutrients. To insure we get all the proper vitamins and minerals it is important that we supplement where necessary. This of course does not mean that we don't use as our first line of defense pure organic healthy foods.

Supplementation however is a complex subject, not very well understood by most medical doctors. We are then left with a myriad of information, some times contradictory.

Not only is it confusing as to what to take for what, but we also don't know the right amounts, or what will mix with what. My firm belief is that when you are adding supplements to your diet it is important to work with a qualified practitioner. Each person is unique as are their needs. Yes, we should take a good multivitamin every day, but adding additional supplements may counteract or eliminate the benefit.

A qualified practitioner will do a case study, looking into not only your physical self, but also your emotional and soulful self. The practitioner realizes that energy (which is all that we are) needs to be balanced on all levels.

Disease comes about because of a deficiency, or disturbance in the flow of energy. Energy to be balanced needs all the important nutrients in the proper amounts. Although we may be able to diagnose our own deficiencies to a degree, it is best to seek out the assistance of someone who has studied and works with supplements. It is also important to get good quality supplements. Many supplements have fillers that can be toxic.

The sale of nutritional supplements is a billion-dollar industry. There are any numbers of books on the subject of supplements and nutrition. Unfortunately, few have sound scientific backing. One of the Books that I highly recommend is *The Real Vitamin and Mineral Book* by Sherri Lieberman. I had the privilege of meeting Sherri as she was a guest on a radio show that I co-host with Dr. Mitchell Ghen. This book is a very informative book about vitamins and minerals. It is a good reference. I believe that the more you know when you begin to work with practitioners the better your questions. This helps the practitioner to assist you in developing a comprehensive program.

Vitamins and mineral are essential to life. We call them micronutrients because compared to proteins, carbohydrates fats and water; we only need a small amount.

Minerals are needed for the proper composition of our body fluids, in bone and blood formation and to maintain healthy nerve function.

For nearly forty years the RDA or recommended daily allowances, set by the United States Food and Nutrition Board have been used as the guideline. The problem is that the guidelines are based upon us getting the nutrients from our foods alone. Since we know that today that is nearly impossible, we may need to supplement.

The RDAs do not ensure optimum health. We cannot always get the nutrients from the foods that we eat and the RDAs do not take into account the individual needs.

Most people simply do not eat a well-balanced diet. According to the National Research Council most of us eat far too much fat, sugar, and simple carbohydrates. We live in a world of fast foods and stress, sometimes making it impossible to eat sensibly, in the right portions, and in a stress-free environment.

In addition, for us to get all the nutrients we need from our diet we would need to consume about 2000 calories per day for a woman and about 3000 calories per day for a man. This is about twice the amount that is allowed on the average reducing diet and it has been estimated that about one-third of America is dieting at any given time.

Even if we are not dieting most of us are trying to maintain our weight and would not be consuming 2000-3000 calories per day. And probably although watching our calories we are not consuming health-enhancing foods.

The nutrient contents of the minerals in our foods fluctuate due to the growing conditions. So, although we could be eating healthy, our fruits and vegetables could be deficient in minerals.

Fruits and vegetables also begin to lose their nutrient content as soon as they are picked, more when cut and still more when cooked or processed.

Perhaps the biggest problem is in the milling of grains. When wheat is processed to flour 65 to 85 percent of the B vitamins are depleted. When rice bran is milled the most nutrition part of the bran is hulled off. Further if the rice is milled into white rice, virtually all the nutrients are lost.

Chemicals and pollutants invade our environment and rob our body of nutrients. Foods such as hot dogs, bacon, ham and bologna are processed with nitrates.

Stress, disease, drugs and aging are factors that determine both the quality of the nutrients we get and the assimilation. When the body works harder it needs more energy.

Studies have shown that as you age your organs tend to function less efficiently. Because digestion and elimination seem to be a problem associated with aging, we may not be getting adequate amounts of nutrient even when eating a sensible diet.

In addition, many diseases associated with aging such as cancer, diabetes, high blood pressure, heart disease and excelled aging have been shown to have nutritional implications.

Inadequate nutrition has been shown to weaken the immune system. Eating a proper diet will help, but we may also need to supplement.

We need to supplement because:
1. We are not meeting the RDAs even if we are eating a proper diet
2. The foods available to us do not contain the amounts of vitamins and minerals they should contain

3. We require higher levels of nutrients due to the constant bombardment of stress
4. Vitamins and minerals are never 100 percent absorbed.

Do we need to supplement? Unfortunately, we do even under the best of conditions. However, it is important to get the best quality supplements and to work with a practitioner who can guide you through the maze.

Remember supplementation means to supplement and is not a substitute for a healthy diet.

CELLULAR RESPIRATION
~ THE KISS OF LIFE

B reath in yoga is considered the kiss of life. It is our first noble inspiration and our last noble expiration. Prana, we know is the force that gives rise to breath and all the energy of the universe. It is the force behind all that exist.

Yoga looks upon the body as having a consciousness as well as three distinct modes of functioning, called the Triune or:
1. The physical body
2. The astral body- the mind
3. The casual body – the soul

Each part of the triune depends upon and supports the other. If one part is out of balance the other two are also out of balance. It is sort of like an atom whose electron gets knocked out of balance creating a free radical that then needs to be countered by an antioxidant. The body and the mind are supported and can be balanced by the foods we eat and the breathes we take. The soul just needs earth energy and the only way it gets it is from the body and the mind. So be careful with what you feed your body and what you let occupy your mind; they are the soul's vehicle and GPS. Keeping the body healthy and the mind clear also requires oxygen.

Oxygen, which is essential to life, is the fuel our cells use to break down and use the nutrients found in our foods. This is called cellular respiration, which is not to be confused with the breathing of oxygen, although the breathing of oxygen is essential to life. Locked inside the whole foods that we eat is the vital element of oxygen. All living things have oxygen cells embedded in them. Our cells need oxygen as an energy source to break down the nutrients from our foods. This is why it is important to eat whole live foods. Plants use photosynthesis to absorb carbon dioxide and sunlight from the air. They convert this energy into oxygen and glucose and this is how plants help us with cellular respiration; they provide us with extra oxygen so we can turn our nutrients into energy.

Anna yoga means making conscious choices about the quantity and quality of the foods we give to our body and our mind. Maya-kosha means the temporary shield that supports our health. That means that we must constantly replenish the body-mind with energy that supports both life and health.

The breath is considered the "kiss of life" It is in a constant exchange of inhale and exhale taking in oxygen and expelling carbon dioxide. Our diet should compliment the "kiss of life, or the taking in of life and the expelling of waste. Our diets should always reflect that which supports and compliments the kiss of life.

THE SENSORY WORLD

Anna yoga like all branches of yoga reminds us to be aware of our attachment to the world through our sensory experience. We experience our world through our senses; however, the senses can get us into trouble. We taste something sweet and immediately the sense of taste wants more. Therefore, we need the consciousness of the intellect to discern, evaluate and decide what we need, what we want and how to satisfy. The senses in and of themselves have no judgment, evaluative, or discretionary faculties. The sense organs of taste, scent, hearing, sight and touch simply sense our world. It is the intellect that establishes what is beneficial and what is not.

When we are immersed in deep thought our senses are still. We can be so deep in thought that we do not hear any sounds around us. It is only when our minds draw us to something through the desire of the sense organs that we attach to objects.

As the senses reach out and attach themselves to things, the mind desires to possess these things. Once the mind possesses them it fears losing them and not possessing them the mind becomes distressed and agitated. An agitated mind is a scattered mind, which dissipates our energy and causes us to experience chaos.

The process of sense withdrawal is used in Anna yoga to direct us away from those things that do us harm and towards those that support life. We learn to draw energies away from objects by turning inward. This is known as detachment.

Through the mastery of the senses the intellectual mind becomes free of emotions and attachment and is free to discern that which is supporting and that which is destructive. The intellect disciplines the senses to stop their cravings and desires. The senses cease to run after external objects. Cravings cease and the mind becomes quiet.

Anna yoga teaches the intellectual conscious choice making of the quiet intellect. It teaches us to quiet the body-mind and make conscious choices about the foods we eat. We learn to quiet the cravings and desires through the understanding and knowledge of what will support and enhance life.

For most humans' life is a painful process of continual ups and downs. This is because they are locked into the possessiveness and continuity of things and cannot adjust to the ever-changing conditions of life. They are unable to release themselves from things because they are unable to control their senses, cravings and desires.

Detachment releases one from the negativity of the mind. It is not a detachment for the objects, but from our reactions to these objects. This means we need to detach from all things, pleasurable and painful, external and internal. Being attached we are caught up in the shackles of bondage and this bondage causes us to have cravings. Cravings grow and can never be satisfied. We always want more.

Cravings cause addictions and addictions cause the mind to be confused. When the mind is confused you lose the power of discernment. When we lose the power of discernment, we lose the meaning and purpose of life, which is to find contentment and happiness. What is life without happiness?

Yoga teaches us that when the five sense organs, as well as the mind and the intellect are passive, we reach a state of inner realization, an understanding of wisdom and a place of peace and serenity.

Regarding sight, studies at Brotheaver National Laboratories, found that when people see their favorite foods the pleasure neurotransmitter, dopamine is released. There is a correlation between addictive behavior and the release of dopamine.

When we talk about taste we generally mean a combination of taste and smell. When people complain about losing their sense of taste, they generally mean they have an impaired sense of smell. With any sensory system the brain must determine not only what the stimulus is, but also what it means. The latter is crucial in terms of taste because it tells the brain whether to swallow, or spit it out. Taste combined with the sense of smell has a strong impact on our thought process, especially when it comes to foods. We appreciate and learn to discriminate foods and drinks based upon both taste and smell.

If asked which sense most people would give up, if they had to eliminate one, most would say smell. Smell however is more important than we might think as it alters the social behavior in most mammals including humans. Pheromones are the odorous chemicals, or scents we all give off. Animals respond sexually to the scent given off by males and females. Even humans to some extend respond to the scents of one another.

Olfactory cells (sense of smell) carry chemical messages to the olfactory bulb which is part of the limbic system of your brain. It is connected to the cerebral cortex and is also made up of the amygdala, the hippocampus and hypothalamus. The hippocampus is the connection to your memory and the hypothalamus is connected to your sense of thirst and hunger. Therefore, the sense of smell has a profound effect on the foods we desire and the foods we eat.

Eating is a sensory experience. It is the awareness of the power of the senses and the ability to withdraw and control that provides the balance needed to make conscious choices about the quality and quantity of the foods we eat.

It is not that we should not embrace, explore, and experience the sensory world. After all it is through the senses that we gain experience and experience brings both knowledge and wisdom. Through withdrawal we learn to become the observer of our lives, consciously guiding the senses towards that which creates the greatest good and serves us well. The discerning mind makes these decisions through the process of learning. Anna yoga teaches us how through our diets we can experience the path of enlightenment. When we choose consciously that which creates the greatest *good,* we discover our inherent nature, which is the balanced rhythm of expansion and contraction.

But what is the greatest good? It is that which supports and enhances life. The purpose of life is to gain wisdom and wisdom is gained through the long learning process of life.

It is the nature of the tongue to appreciate taste and the nature of the nose to appreciate smell. No matter the person, that which taste sweet, taste sweet. The tongue cannot behave against its inherent nature. The goal of Anna yoga is not to change the senses, but to transcend them and experience non-attachment.

The sense of taste is responsible, as are the other senses, for desires and repulsions. Although it is the nature of the senses to function, they must not be allowed to function in an uncontrolled manner. We should always remain unattached, which does not mean indifference. Detachment means the ability to release yourself from emotionality, which impairs your sense of balance and destroys your discerning powers.

The average person by his very nature becomes locked into the sense organs. They miss the ultimate connection with reality by believing that what is experienced through the senses is the only reality. Through the sense organs we perceived the material world, but it is this perception that we confuse for our true nature. We begin to feel that we are what we perceive. If we perceive we are miserable over a certain amount of time we become that misery.

Anna yoga teaches us to focus on the sensory world and learn through the process. The process teaches us to focus on that, which gives us the greatest good so that what we taste, we truly taste and what we smell we truly smell. With this we become one with the essence of what we eat and drink and this supports our health. This self-control then becomes a natural state of being.

Yoga teaches that when we train the sense organs, the mind and the intellect to become quiet, we reach a state of sense withdrawal. This does not mean that the senses cease to function, but rather that we train them to pull away from their cravings and desires and become somewhat suspended. We become the passive observer of all that we do, thus wisely choosing that which does no harm and does the greatest good.

Sense withdrawal leads us beyond the everyday states of wakefulness, dreaming and sleep into an inner state where the soul finds peace and contentment no matter what the circumstances.

METABOLIC BALANCE EXERCISE

B uild strength and established balance, while increasing your metabolism.

Seek balance in all things and in all things find balance.

Anna yoga promotes the ideals of a long and radiant life through the use of a healthy and proper diet combined with physical exercise. If we wish to increase our life energy we must support the body-mind with nutrients and activities that promote these ideals.

The problem with being over weight may not be body weight in pounds as much as the amount of body fat. The problem with most people, who are over weight, is that their metabolism is sluggish. This in part is due to poor nutrition and lack of exercise. Remember most of the calories people consume, however are not used for exercise, but used for basal metabolism, the energy that is used to constantly monitor body temperature. And metabolic rates do vary depending upon a number of factors, including genetics, diet and exercise.

When researchers studied the effects of exercise without dietary restrictions, they found that those who did regular exercise lost 10 to 15 precent of body weight without dieting. Researchers actually found that dieting alone actually reduced metabolic rate. That's because exercise builds body muscle and muscles burn more calories than fat. Lean muscle mass actually makes it easier to lose and maintain weight. The research was based upon aerobic exercise and weight lifting.

Yoga, however is gaining momentum as a great way to build muscle mass and increase metabolism.

When it comes to metabolism two of the most recognized forms of exercise are aerobics and weight lifting. Aerobics builds cardiovascular strength, which improves our breathing, heart rate and burns calories, but it does not build muscle strength like weight training. This does not mean we don't want to do aerobic exercise. It simply means that to build general overall physical health through exercise we need to focus on endurance, strength, and flexibility. Weight training provides the strength and yoga provides both strength and flexibility. The ideal is a combination of all three forms of exercise.

The aging process presents us with two health problems that can be easily reduced through weight bearing exercise. One of course is osteoporosis and the second is what is known as Sarcopenia, or the age-related term for the decline in lean muscle mass. Osteoporosis has to do with loss of bone mass. Numerous studies have shown that a healthy diet rich in calcium and magnesium combined with weight bearing/resistance exercise is the best preventative measure against osteoporosis.

Sarcopenia cannot be reverses but can be controlled with regular weight bearing exercises. With sarcopenia your body may stay the same weight as you age, but the lean muscle mass begins to atrophy; meaning the muscle slowly erodes and is replaced with fat. To slow the process weight bearing and yoga are the best forms of exercise.

Constant dieting can make sarcopenia worse because most short-term diets deplete muscle mass and actually increase fat. Since lean muscle burns more calories that fat, dieting can actually reduce the body's ability to burn fat. With less lean muscle your metabolism drops and your weight not only comes back faster, but it is also harder to lose.

Be patient and diligent with any exercise program you incorporate into your life. Consistency is the key to success. Don't look to lose weight quickly, or to quickly build muscle mass. It took time to get where you're at and it will take time to get where you're going. The choices you make are about lifestyle. And like everything in life it is a long learning process that involves time and commitment.

In yoga we use the term greed to mean we reach beyond our limits to the degree that we injure ourselves. When you injure yourself, you must retract and heal and thus inhibit yourself from expanding. Always practice non-greed and non-harm.

> *"On with the dance, let joy be unconfined is my motto,*
> *whether there is any dance to dance or any joy unconfined."*
> *~ Mark Twain ~*

FOOD FACTS

With a plethora of nutrition information available, it is sometimes difficult to get answers to the simple questions regarding a healthy diet. I am constantly asked by my students and clients questions about various foods and whether they are healthy or not. The following questions and answers will help you to gain an understanding of the foods that are included in the yogi diet. We are seeking to find balance and health, so remember the yogi diet means that we seek to do no harm. In doing so it is important to make good food choices.

Before we can put together a healthy eating plan, we need to gain knowledge. Knowledge and experience bring us wisdom. We can gain knowledge from reading and studying, but it is through experience that we develop wisdom. Therefore, yoga teaches us to take the knowledge we have learned and experience it through life. As in the laws of karma yoga, we find a need and fill it. So, this section is about gaining knowledge. Take this knowledge and then apply it to your life and you will gain the wisdom and understanding of what it means to find an inner sense of peace and self love.

True understanding comes from loving something with such a passion that you seek to learn all you can about this something. What better something to love than yourself and your health? Your body-mind is the vehicle and GPS of your soul and since our journey is to find wisdom, the journey is much better served with a strong body, clean mind, and pure heart.

Paracelsus, an ancient alchemist who is often credited as the father of modern chemistry wrote:

"He, who knows nothing, loves nothing. He who can do nothing, understands nothing. He who understands nothing is worthless. But he, who understands, loves, notices, sees... The more knowledge inherent in a thing, the greater the love...anyone who imagines that all fruit ripens at the same time as the strawberries, knows nothing of the grapes."

Q : WHAT IS A BALANCED DIET?

A balanced diet should include an adequate amount of all the food groups. Most Americans are familiar with the food pyramid as the guideline for a balanced and healthy diet. The United States Department of Agriculture Food Guide Pyramid was introduced decades ago. Although it does provide a basic guideline it is quite heavy in carbohydrates and does not distinguish between simple and complex carbohydrates.

A healthy balanced diet means to get the right balance of complex carbohydrates, protein and fats to avoid the risk for chronic disease. Unfortunately, the USDA pyramid not only promotes too many carbohydrates, but also promotes three servings of dairy and too many servings of fruits per day.

Scientific studies see (www.oldwayspt.org) have shown that the Mediterranean, Asian and Vegetarian pyramids may in fact be a healthier approach to a balanced diet. This is because they promote less meat and more of a plant-based diet, as well as the use of good fats such as olive oil and minimal amounts of dairy.

Basically, a balanced diet should include the food groups of complex carbohydrates (6- 11 servings per day), protein – 0.8 to 1.2 grams per kilogram (2.2) of body weight per day (mostly fish and plant based), and The American Heart Association recommends no more than 30 percent total fat per day; with no more than 10 percent being saturated fat. Dairy should be limited to a serving of yogurt or kefir as most dairy products produce mucus in the body. We should be getting five to seven servings of vegetables per day and two to four servings of fruit per day.

Anna-maya-kosha yoga teaches everything in moderation. It's ok to have the occasional dessert and the occasional drink, as long as you keep things in balance and remember to do no harm. Living a balanced and healthy lifestyle is a personal decision. Choose to eat healthy for yourself with love and devotion.

Q : IS THE PROTEIN DIET GOOD OR BAD AND HOW MUCH PROTEIN DO WE REALLY NEED?

Dr Atkins is famous for the protein diet. Many people claim to have lost weight on the diet; however, studies show that most people put the weight back on. How can a diet that promotes heavy protein and heavy fat and almost eliminates, fruits, vegetables and complex carbohydrates be good for you? Again, scientific studies show that a healthy and balanced diet that includes the right amount of all the food groups supports health.

According to an article in the ACE Fitness Matters magazine September/October 2002, there are some divided opinions over the amount of protein needed. However, some general recommendations are given.

Proteins are essential and cannot be synthesized by the body. This means we must obtain the proteins from our foods. Proteins are used to support, transport and provide nutrients to the body. Proteins strengthen the immune system and regulate our metabolism. Other proteins do the work of building bones, ligaments, tendons and organs. In terms of exercise, proteins function in the growth and repair of muscle tissues.

Protein requirements depend upon the level of activity and fitness level of the individual. An unconditioned person needs 0.8 grams of protein per kilogram (2.2 pounds) of body weight per day. Those doing a regular exercise program of 45-60 minutes of aerobics and/or weight training per day need to take in about 1.2 - 1.4 grams per day per kilogram of body weight.

Many experts believe that the timing of protein is crucial to replacing fuel and repairing muscles. Data suggest that it is important to get both complex carbohydrates and protein after a workout. Experts advise that we should get 1.5 grams of carbohydrates, per body weight, within a half hour after exercising and then consume the same amount about two hours later with 1 gram of protein. In other words, eat carbohydrates and proteins within an hour or two after exercise. Men and women should follow the same measured guidelines for protein consumption.

Are some protein sources better than others? Experts agree that we need to get complete proteins, which are found in fish, eggs, chicken, beef, tofu and dairy. However incomplete proteins such as nuts, grains, legumes and vegetables can be combined to make complete proteins, which supports a plant-based diet.

Recent studies indicate that whey a milk by-product is a fully absorbable protein source, followed by egg whites, red meat, poultry, fish, dairy products and plant proteins. Combining proteins seems to provide the best source of getting a complete and balance protein allotment. Over consumption of red meat can lead to elevated cholesterol so it is best to tailor your diet to your own needs, vary your proteins and practice moderation. Remember you know your body better than anyone.

Q : CARBOHYDRATES — WHAT IS THE DIFFERENCE BETWEEN COMPLEX AND SIMPLE?

All carbohydrates regardless of their source are metabolized into glucose, which is sugar. Increased levels of sugar in your body will signal the body to produce insulin, which is the hormone that signals the body to store fat. Both the amount and the type of carbohydrates you eat affect the storage of fat.

Basically, the simpler the carbohydrate that greater the amount of insulin it will trigger. Simple carbohydrates are refined foods such as white flour, sugar, breads, cakes, cookies, pastas, candy, and other desserts and snack foods such as chips and crackers. Complex carbohydrates are whole grains and natural whole foods such as fresh fruits and vegetables.

If you want to maintain a healthy balanced diet, and also lose weight, as well as eliminate that spare tire around the middle, switch from simple carbohydrates to complex carbohydrates. Complex carbohydrates can also have a profound effects upon your moods.

Q : GOOD FATS OR BAD FATS?

Our bodies need fat for functional reasons including energy production and organ insulation. However, it is often confusing as to what a so-called "good" fat is and what is a so called 'bad" fat.

The fats most often found in food are called triglycerides, which mean three (tri) fatty acid chains joined with half a sugar molecule. You probably think of them as bad cause your doctor often warns against too high a triglyceride count.

Some triglycerides are made from saturated fats; however not all saturated fats are bad for you. Saturated fats are found in meat, butter, milk, cheese, ice cream, chocolate and palm oils. These fats stay solid at room temperature and therefore generally speaking are not good for the body. However, one saturated fat that is considered good for the body is stearic acid, found in meat. A small study done by Pennsylvania State University suggests that a diet high in stearic acid may reduce high levels of bad cholesterol. Unfortunately beef also has high levels of bad saturated fats, so a little beef goes a long way!

Unsaturated fats, which tend to be liquid at room temperature, come in two types, polyunsaturated and monounsaturated. The fatty acids coming from these two fats hold the cells together. Monounsaturated fats found in olive oil and canola oil are good, but not as good as polyunsaturated fats.

Even if you eat a fat free diet your body can produce saturated and monounsaturated fats. However, if you don't eat adequate amounts of polyunsaturated fats (approximately 4 to 6 percent of daily calories), you could develop deficiencies. Humans cannot convert other fats into polyunsaturated fats so you must receive them through the diet. That's why polyunsaturated fats are also known as essential fatty acids. The most important essential fatty acid is linoleic, an omega 6, most common in seed oils such as corn, sunflower, cottonseed and safflower. Primrose oil and black currant oil also contain high levels of linoleic acid. Preliminary studies have indicated that omega 6 may help to reduce the symptoms of premenstrual syndrome and data suggest that it stimulates the metabolism, and thus helps to burn calories. Primrose, borage and black currant oils are suggested. Flaxseed oil is also recommended.

The other essential fatty acid is linolenic, an omega 3, found primarily in fish such as salmon, mackerel, sardines, herring, anchovies, and tuna, and in nuts (especially almonds) and canola oil and soybean oil and in flax seed. Your body relies upon these two essential fatty acids to perform the metabolic function of keeping a healthy immune system. It is called the yin (omega 6 – to push) and the yang (omega 3 - to pull back) of your metabolic system.

Man made trans fats, which are the hydrogenated fats, are the margarines, shortening, and fats found in most packaged baked goods, candy and crackers. Trans fats tend to "gum" up our inner body. Researchers believe there is a link between breast cancer and heart attack and high levels of hydrogenated fat.

Cholesterol is by far the most notorious fat formed by the liver. You need it to insulate your nerves and maintain cell membranes. LDL is the so called "bad "cholesterol and HDL is the so called "good" cholesterol.

The body manufactures HDL. It is crucial to the production of sex hormones, as well as to liver function, and the production of vitamin

D. Cholesterol travels from the liver through the blood stream where it is delivered to the cells. The cells take what they need and the excess remains in the blood stream. When we eat a diet that is high in LDL cholesterol, the body has an excess of cholesterol, which cannot be removed by the HDL and therefore tends to clog the arteries. When the diet is not high in fat the HDL carries excess cholesterol back to the liver for elimination.

Americans typically eat a high saturated fat diet and lead sedentary lifestyles. This is why dietary cholesterol usually gets cast into the bad category. Our bodies can make enough cholesterol, without the need for dietary cholesterol. When we eat excess meat, dairy and processed foods we risk overloading the system.

The sensible way to keep serum fats within a safe range is to eat very little meat and dairy products, avoid processed foods and consume fiber such as whole grains, fruits and vegetables.

Olive oil has been shown to be relatively heart healthy although experts advise to consume in moderation. We don't know how much fat is good for you, but what we do know is that cutting down on saturated fats, reading food labels and exercising can help to reduce high levels of cholesterols.

Experts also advise to cut back on sugar and alcohol, as well as reduce stress levels. Coffee should also be moderated.

Q : WHAT ABOUT SUGAR AND SUGAR SUBSTITUTES?

The average American consumes about 60 pounds of sugar per year and favors carbonated drinks to other drinks when not consuming 2.6 gallons of alcoholic beverages per year, both of which are high in sugar.

More diseases have been linked to eating sugar than to any other aspect of nutrition. One of the most important characteristics of sugar is that it is a simple carbohydrate that cannot be digested, assimilated, or utilized by the body without the help of other nutrients that must be provided from nutritious foods in your diet, or from nutrients that are stored in the blood and bones. If the diet is deficient in nutritious foods the body cannot process the sugar.

Sugar also prohibits the ability of the white blood cells in your immune system to keep the growth of bacteria in the body; in check. The effects of sugar last for about four hours, so if you eat sugar for breakfast, lunch and dinner your body is constantly vulnerable to a misbalance in bacteria and this weakens your immune system. Over consumption of sugar (sucrose) if likely to aggravate if not cause, tooth decay, diabetes, hypoglycemia, coronary disease, obesity, ulcers, high blood pressure, vaginal yeast infections, osteoporosis and malnutrition.

Fructose is often used as a substitute for sucrose. Although it is derived from fruit, it is generally refined like sucrose and comes in the form of corn syrup, which is a simple carbohydrate.

Refined white sugar is the most heavily contaminated of the sucrose sweeteners having been sprayed with multiple pesticides, processed over natural gas flame and chemically bleached. Black strap molasses, brown sugar, corn syrup, and dextrose are other forms of sucrose that have not been chemically treated.

Artificial sweeteners such as saccharin and aspartame have potential health risk. The problem is over consumption, which is easy with aspartame being used in nearly every food product from breakfast cereals to vitamins pills.

Aspartame contains phenylalanine, which in high dosages is toxic to the brain. People experience headaches, depression, mood swings, high blood pressure, and insomnia, and behavior problems as a result of chemical changes in the brain caused by sweeteners.

Instead of sugar eat naturally sweet foods such as whole fruits, or use one of the many sweeteners that do not rely upon sucrose as their sweetening agent.

Q : WHAT ABOUT CALCIUM AND OSTEOPOROSIS?

Calcium is an important mineral that is used for nerve transmission, blood clotting and the activation of the enzymes used for fat and protein digestion, as well as the formation of bones and teeth. Calcium also aids in the absorption of nutrients, especially vitamin B-12. Our bodies contain approximately 2 ½ pounds of calcium, 99 percent of which is stored in our bones and teeth. The remaining 1 percent is distributed throughout our body in the blood stream and fluids surrounding the cells.

Normally, if there is enough calcium in the diet the blood and bone calcium stay balanced. However, if there is a deficiency then the body reacts by taking calcium from the bones and using it in the blood to keep the heart beating regularly. The body will always choose to maintain certain levels of blood calcium over bone calcium. This is accomplished by a complex system involving the parathyroid hormone, which increases blood calcium and decrease potassium.

Calcium intake is clearly a major factor in the development of osteoporosis, however other elements in the diet and lifestyle factors need to be considered. Approximately 20 million American women and 2 million American men are affected by osteoporosis. Women are more likely to develop osteoporosis because they make less bone and lose it at a greater rate than men. But men are now accounting for about one fifth the cost of osteoporosis.

Hormonal changes in both men and women can cause osteoporosis. The sharp decline in estrogen following menopause is one major factor. One of estrogens roles is to incorporate calcium into the bones. In men low testosterone levels can lead to osteoporosis.

For proper assimilation calcium needs magnesium, iron, manganese, phosphorous, Vitamin A, C, D, and F. Most experts will tell you to take calcium with magnesium. Phosphorous is another mineral that needs to be considered. Most experts advise a ratio of calcium to phosphorous should be 1:1. In other words we should take in an equal amount of phosphorous to calcium. If phosphorous intake is too high, it impairs the absorption of calcium, as well as increases the amount drawn from the bones.

If our diets contain phosphorous rich foods such as meats, soft drinks and food additives we may be getting too much phosphorous. Studies have linked high protein and high fat diets with the loss of calcium from the body.

A proper diet, exercise and a little sunshine help to keep bones healthy and strong. Dairy foods are rich in calcium; however, they are also high in fat. If you are eliminating dairy from your diet, eat non-fat yogurt and kefir a liquid type yogurt. Both are rich in calcium, low in fat and help to keep the good flora (bacteria) in the gut and intestines. Canned salmon and sardines are excellent calcium choices. So are leafy greens, clams, oysters, shrimp, kale, broccoli, soybeans and tofu.

Don't use antacids as calcium supplements. Many contain aluminum; a heavy metal that can have adverse effects on your health. It is best to get your calcium through your diet and through proper supplementation.

The US Department of Agriculture conducted a study on the effects of the mineral boron on postmenopausal women and osteoporosis. The results of the study suggested that boron works much like estrogen to prevent bone loss. As little as three milligrams of boron can double levels of circulating estrogen. Boron is found in strawberries, asparagus, figs, poppy seeds, broccoli, pears, cherries, tomatoes, dandelions, apples, beets, apricots, currants, and parsley, and cumin seed.

Every man and woman over the age of 50 should get a bone density test. They should also be getting about 1000 to 1200 mg of calcium per day Also get about 400 to 800 mg of magnesium per day. Get some sunshine, which produces vitamin D, or take 400IU of D per day. Reduce consumption of sugar, salt, alcohol, caffeine, protein and soft drinks. Do resistant exercise such as lifting weights and yoga, which is an excellent resistant exercise program.

Q : IS SOY AND TOFU REALLY GOOD FOR YOU?

All soybean products such as tofu and soybean milk are complete proteins. This means that soybean products provide all the essential amino acids. Complete proteins are essential to life. They provide the structure for all living things. Proteins such as beans, cheese, nuts, and wheat are not complete proteins and must be eaten in combination to make a complete protein. Soy products are therefore an excellent choice for a vegetarian or meatless diet. Soy is also an isoflavonoid, and a phytoestrogen. Isoflavonoids act as antioxidants and phytoestrogens provide the body with a natural plant-based estrogen. Together they work to reduce the risk of breast cancer and prostate cancer. Natural plant-based estrogens can be effective in helping a woman through menopause. Studies have shown that Asian women on an Asian diet have less severe menopausal symptoms and less breast cancer. It is believed that this is related to soy in the diet.

Soybeans are high in two estrogen-like plant compounds, genistein and daidzein. Both of these prevent the body from taking up the more harmful estrogen that is circulating in your blood. When your body produces too much estrogen these phytoestrogens work to reduce, or block the uptake, and when estrogen level is low they work to increase the production. This may explain in part why soy has been effective in the treatment of PMS and menopause (estrogen levels drop premenstrual and menopausal).

So, what is the down side of soy? Soybean products contain certain enzyme inhibitors and should be consumed in moderation. Over consumption could cause digestive problems. This simply means a constant diet of soy "everything" could be hazardous to your health. Eating a soy meal everyday, or several times a week is not going to hurt you; however, eating soy constantly may have an effect on your digestion. Anything in excess especially at the compromise of other things has the potential to create problems. The American Medical Journal has reported out that soy, or the isoflavonoid genistein, may help to decrease cancer, improve night vision, and act as an antioxidant. So, add soy to your diet!

Q : ARE NUTS GOOD FOR YOU?

Many people in early Biblical times owned olive, or fig tree groves, but the so-called "richer people" also had almonds, walnuts and pistachios. Walnuts were thought to bring good luck and good health. The tradition of nuts as a healing food continued into the Middle Ages. Walnuts were considered so powerful that they were included in a prescription to ward off even the dreaded black plague.

One of the reasons nuts are so nutritious and are rated so highly is that they are rich in important minerals such as potassium, zinc, copper, iron, calcium, and magnesium, and phosphorous. All nuts also contain protease inhibitors, which appear to be natural cancer blockers.

Nuts are also loaded with polyphenols, another substance that researchers now believe help to tackle cancer cells.

The oil found in walnuts, is one of the "good" polyunsaturated fats and tend to lower cholesterol levels.

The ancient tradition of giving nuts as offerings of peace and goodwill has been carried down for centuries. It is the health giving and healing aspect of nuts that serve to provide us with a food that has both health and goodwill meaning.

Seeds should also be considered, and also fall into the same category as nuts. Sesame seeds, pumpkin seeds and sunflower seeds all provide important minerals and proteins. Sesame seeds are a great source of fiber as well as essential fatty acids.

Q : WHAT ABOUT MOLASSES, HONEY AND MAPLE SYRUP AS SUBSTITUTES FOR SUGAR?

All three are far better choices than white sugar, however all three are also high in calories.

Black strap molasses is actually unprocessed sucrose. Although it is a sucrose sugar it is high in iron and often used as a tonic for energy. See the recipe section for yogi tonic.

Maple syrup is sap from the maple tree. The Government actually regulates that maple syrup (to be called maple syrup) be made from maple sap syrup. It is also sucrose, but again has not been processed like white sugar.

Honey is the nectar of the bees. The name comes from the Hebrew word that means, "enchant". Long before it was used as a culinary sweetener, honey was valued for its many healing properties. Honey is generally the least chemically contaminated sweetener because bees exposed to pesticides usually don't make it back to the hive.

An ancient Egyptian scroll lists more than 500 remedies using honey as a primary ingredient. Honey rubbed into wounds was a rapid and effective healer. In 1979 a British study found that surgical wounds healed faster when treated with honey. Honey kills dangerous bacteria both on the inside and outside of the body.

Honey has been used to treat asthma, allergies, sore throats, upset digestive tract and insomnia. Honey can lull you to sleep because it is a complex carbohydrate containing natural sugars. Biochemists know that our bodies burn chemical substances called serotonin. Serotonin relaxes us and helps us to sleep. Complex carbohydrates such as honey help the brain to produce serotonin.

Honey also provides a healthful pick-me-up. The bees that produce it have predigested the glucose and fructose in honey. These sugars are quickly and easily absorbed into the human digestive tract, and they have an overall soothing effect. Honey is a health food but should be used sparingly because again it is high in calories.

Look for honey that has not been heated and has been produced by beekeepers that do not feed their bees refined sugar or use harmful pesticides.

Q : COFFEE – IS IT GOOD OR IS IT BAD?

The bad: it's a stimulant that gives you the jitters, raises blood pressure, making you edgy, and causes an acidic digestive system. Coffee consumption can promote the excretion of calcium from the bones. Drinking decaffeinated coffee may be worse than drinking non decaffeinated as the solvents used to remove the caffeine contain cancer-causing chemicals. The good: caffeine is the most commonly used mind-altering drug in the world. Research indicate that moderate amounts may help to maintain mental health as we age. Coffee is also a good source of antioxidants and has been shown to enhance a good workout. Its smells good and taste good, but be aware of additives and fancy drinks that add sugar and calories. Moderation is the key – 1-2 cups per day.

Q : WHAT ABOUT GREEN TEA?

Although green tea is a stimulant and does have caffeine, it is less acidic than coffee and is rich in antioxidants. Studies have shown that green tea increases metabolism and that the heating effect of tea (which also includes herbal teas) helps the body to burn fat after a meal. Studies have shown that the antioxidants in green tea may be effective as a preventative to memory loss associated with aging.

Q : WHAT ABOUT ALCOHOL CONSUMPTION? IS IT TRUE THAT RED WINE AND BEER ARE GOOD FOR YOU?

Is it any wonder that we are all confused about the effects of alcohol on our health? One study says alcohol is good for us and another says it impairs. Both however do make the claim that moderation is the key. Alcohol is mostly simple sugar and beer is a simple carbohydrate (sugar). Red wine however seems to be the secret as to why Europeans have less heart disease. Red wine is loaded with flavonoids and antioxidants, which have been shown to both help, oxidize "bad" LDL cholesterol and improve circulation, which also seems to have an effect on the prevention of Alzheimer's disease and dementia. Red wine is also a great source of quercetin, an antioxidant and anti-inflammatory substance that kills cancer cells and controls blood sugar.

However, the conclusion is that alcohol should only be consumed in moderation; one glass a day.

For those who don't want to consume alcohol, grape seed extract has been shown to have the same effects as red wine. Scientists found that grape seed extract has flavonoids that initiate the release of nitric oxide. Nitric oxide is found in the blood and is used by the body for circulation. Viagra uses nitric oxide to improve blood flow to the sexual organs. Take two 300 milligrams of grape seed oil per day.

Q : WHAT ABOUT SALT, IS IT BAD?

There is a difference in salt. First there is ordinary table salt, which studies have shown can raise your blood pressure, as well as cause you to retain water. There is also Celtic and "hand harvested" sea salt.

Celtic sea salt is probably better than ordinary salt because table salt is almost pure sodium and its sodium that affects blood pressure. Unlike sea salt, Celtic salt contains as many as 50 minerals, including potassium and magnesium.

Experts now believe that low levels of potassium and magnesium are just as much to blame for high blood pressure as too much dietary sodium. Recent research shows that adequate amounts of magnesium and potassium have been shown to lower blood pressure.

Also, these sea salts taste better. Gray salt form Brittany France, gets its flavor from clay. Sicilian salts have a sweeter flavor that's baked in by the Mediterranean sun. Utah sea salt comes from ancient, dry seabeds in the southern part of the United States.

If you must use salt, choose sea salt with its mineral content and great taste.

Q : WHAT ABOUT POTASSIUM?

Our cells contain more potassium than any other mineral. It is essential in maintaining fluid balance within the cells and for the enzymatic reactions taking place within them. Potassium is used for nerve transmission, contraction of muscles and hormone secretion. There is a section of our brain that is essential to take care of fatty products. It's called the "sex brain." If it becomes weakened due to efficiencies, the system cannot efficiently utilize fats and oils.

There is a certain substance called neurolin, which is needed by the brain and nerves. When the sex brain is weak neurolin cannot be assimilated and memorization suffers. The arachnoids membrane of the spinal cord and brain normally secrete the fatty substance needed by the brain, spinal fluid and male generative fluids. If there is a lack of potassium in the system, this important substance is not secreted.

There is growing evidence that low levels of potassium are associated with high blood pressure and cardiovascular disease. In a research study conducted on rats, it was determined that rats supplemented with potassium suffered a 2 percent rate of fatal strokes, as compared with 83 percent in the non-supplemented group.

Low sodium, high fiber and balanced potassium are recommended for reducing blood pressure and the risk of stroke. Foods that increase potassium levels are dairy, fish, fruits, vegetables and grains. However, fruits such as bananas have a relatively low amount of retainable potassium so you would need to eat an enormous amount to get your potassium.

Potassium acts as a body cleanser by converting fats into the proper compounds for the body to process effectively. Improper processing of fats may result in diseases such as rheumatism, high blood pressure and heart disease.

Q : I'VE HEARD SEA VEGETABLES ARE GOOD FOR YOU. WHAT ARE THEY AND WHY ARE THEY GOOD?

Sea vegetables are delicious health building plants harvested from the sea. The familiar ones are kelp and dulse and the seaweeds found in miso soup and in sushi. Sea vegetables contain an extensive range of organic minerals and trace elements necessary for good health. Generally, mineral concentrations are much higher in sea vegetables than land vegetables. Brown vegetables such as kelp are an excellent source of iodine.

Iodine is an essential component of the hormone produced by the thyroid gland, which regulate metabolism. Iodine helps to regulated both an under active and an over active thyroid. The RDA recommends 150mcg/day.

The primary role of iodine is to regulate cellular oxidation. The thyroid hormone accelerates cellular reactions, increases oxygen consumption and basal metabolism, and influences growth and development and energy metabolism.

Studies do indicate that too much iodine may induce thyroid disease, so again everything in moderation. Too much would be about 10 times the daily recommendation. With any kind of disease always check with your primary caregiver before making changes.

Sea vegetables have the ideal potassium to sodium ratio: 2.4:1. A ¼ ounce serving of kelp contains twice the potassium of a banana. They are also an excellent source of balanced calcium and magnesium, as well as, iron, iodine, chromium, vitamin K and small amounts of quality protein.

Research from Japan (the people with greatest longevity and highest consumption of sea vegetables) suggest that sea vegetables have anti-tumor, anti-coagulant, hypo-cholesteric, anti-bacterial, anti-viral and anti-parasitic effects.

Used daily in moderate amounts sea vegetables can be a wonderful addition to your diet. Eating sushi combines both seas vegetables and fish to give your diet both the omega 3 and omega 6 essential fatty acids. For organic quality sea vegetables, visit www.seaveg.com, Maine Coast Sea vegetables. Tell them Doctor Lynn sent you!

Q : IS YOGURT A GOOD SOURCE OF CALCIUM AND WHAT IS THIS PRODUCT CALLED KEFIR?

Plain non-fat organic yogurt is a rich source of calcium and also known for keeping the good flora (bacteria) in the intestinal tract. Although not directly mentioned by name in the Bible, tradition says an Angel promised Abraham that he would live a long life if he ate the biblical version of yogurt. He lived to be 175 years! Yogurt is included in many diets of the Middle East and the Mediterranean.

Dr Elias Metchnikoff conducted experiments at the Pasteur Institute in Paris France and reported that yogurt helped to prevent heart disease. People, he noted who ate large amounts of yogurt seldom became senile and the natural deterioration of the body slowed down. In other words, yogurt eaters seemed to hold off old age.

Research has shown that yogurt culture in the intestinal tract target E. coli bacteria and it helps to maintain a normal balance between good and bad bacteria in the body. With all the good bacteria in yogurt it is a natural antibiotic known to head off disease.

Yogurt also has lots of natural fatty hormonal substances called prostaglandins E-2, which protect the stomach lining against irritants and is the basis of new, but synthetic ulcer medication. Yogurt also lowers LDL while raising the good cholesterol HDL. Recently evidence has been cited that yogurt, or the acidophilus content is a powerful anticancer food. It seems to be effective in preventing colon cancer.

Kefir is like yogurt, but more of a liquid with a tart and refreshing taste. Kefir experts believe has more therapeutic value than yogurt. Its very active yeast and bacteria provide more nutritional value that yogurt as they excel in digesting the foods you eat and in keeping the colon clean and healthy.

Adding a starter culture to milk and gently heating it to a certain temperature makes yogurt. To make kefir, the starter is mixed with grains and cultured at room temperature for 24 hours. Without heating involved important enzymes are not destroyed.

Kefir keeps the small and large intestines clean and free of parasites. Once in the large intestine the beneficial bacteria create lactic acid that balances your blood Ph levels. In this environment parasites cannot survive.

With its 2.5 alcohol content (yeast) kefir is actually alkaline forming in the body making the overall quality of the blood slightly more alkaline. This balanced environment provides a healthy site for friendly bacteria to grow.

Kefir is a complete protein with all the essential amino acids. Your body requires protein to heal and the body must have adequate amounts of minerals to properly digest the protein. Kefir provides essential minerals such as calcium, magnesium and phosphorous which is also important for carbohydrate and fat utilization.

Kefir is a good source of tryptophan the precursor to the production of serotonin the neurochemical that causes us to feel calm. It may reduce levels of depression and insomnia as its conversion is aided by B6, which is also abundant in kefir. Some people call kefir "Nature's Prozac"

Kefir also provides the B vitamins such as B-12, folic acid and B5 pantothenic acid, as well as biotin a coenzyme that assist in the unitization of fatty acids and carbohydrates.

Kefir is an excellent source of B12 the longevity vitamin. B12 is necessary for normal metabolism of nerve tissue and for red blood cell formation. B12 builds immunity and is used to increase energy. It works in conjunction with folic acid to synthesize choline (a fat and cholesterol dissolver). It helps regulate kidney, liver and gallbladder functions.

Kefir also aids in the production of DNA and RNA the body's genetic material. B 12 needs to be combined with calcium during absorption and kefir provides for that.

After taking antibiotic it is essential to restore the good flora in the intestines. Kefir is useful in restoring the balance in your body.
Studies have shown that a diet of cultured foods such as raw cultured vegetables, kefir, yogurt, and miso are key to a generally healthy diet. I would recommend adding kefir to your diet. I believe it has a greater

value than yogurt and has a great taste. Buy the organic plain kefir found in health food stores. See the recipe section of this book and also the detoxify section for ways to add kefir.

Q : HOW MUCH WATER SHOULD I DRINK?

Drink at least eight glasses of water per day, but not with meals as water dilutes the digestive enzymes. If you do drink water at mealtime add lemon, which is a purifier. You should drink water at room temperature as icy cold-water shocks the system. Most of your water should be drank the first half of the day to make up for the fluids you missed at night.

If drinking water is a problem eat plenty of melons, which are a good source of mineral water, as well as flavor your water with herbal teas and fruits.

It is essential to drink plenty of water when you are detoxifying the body. This helps to flush out the toxins and keep you hydrated. When you eat a lot of fiber you need water to help you keep the colon clean and prevent constipation. You should also drink plenty of water when you exercise and immediately afterwards.

If you are feeling tired and lethargic it could be a sign that you are dehydrated. Fatigue can happen because we are not getting enough oxygen to the brain. Water helps the transport system to deliver oxygen rich blood to the brain. Water is essential for carrying oxygen and nutrients to the muscle so exercising without it causes one to tire easily.

So everyday drink plenty of pure clean water and eat fruits and vegetables with high water contents such as melons and greens.

Q : I LOVE CHOCOLATE — IS IT THAT BAD FOR YOU?

Nothing, except for cigarettes drugs and other poisons are bad for you in moderation. In fact, chocolate can be good for you providing it's the right kind of chocolate.

Dark rich, pure chocolate is actually high in polyphenols; plant chemicals found in wine and fruit that are potent antioxidants. The American Journal of Clinical Nutrition shows that polyphenols help stop artery - clogging clots from forming.

Chocolate is usually high in fat and sugar and high in calories. Choose dark organic chocolate but remember everything in moderation.

Q : HOW MUCH FIBER SHOULD I HAVE IN MY DIET?

Dr. Dennis Burkitt a British surgeon studied an east African village for many years. He found a non-existence of obesity, diabetes and colon cancer, as well as other Western culture dietary disease. What he discovered was a diet high in fresh vegetables and fruits and coarse grains. The bran from the grains were highly waste absorbent, increasing the bulk in the bowel and speeding up elimination time.

Speeding up the transit time reduces gas and putrification, more fats and cholesterol are removed from the body, and toxins are removed from the bowels, and muscular strength is improved.

One of the biggest problems in our Western culture is constipation. This is in part due to a diet that is high in sugar and processed and refined foods. When the bowels are not emptied of toxic material, bacteria grows and the result is a diseased and toxic body. Keep in mind that the same blood that circulates the bowels also circulated the brain. If the blood circulating is toxic, it effects our mental processing as well as physical health.

Foods that is high in fiber act as scrubbing agents to clean the walls of the intestines. Whole foods such as fruits and vegetables, nuts, seeds and whole grains contain bulk and fiber.

Q : ARE SOUPS A GOOD DIET FOOD?

Soup to most of us is a comforting food. Studies have also shown that soup can be a great weight loss food. Soup is filling and if it is broth based and low fat its also lower in calories.

In a study of 500 people, the soup eaters ate fewer calories per day and ended up losing weight. This weight loss, researchers believe is due to bulk and weight of the soup, which are key to satisfying hunger.

If you are going to buy soup, try to buy organic soups that you find in the health food store. These will not have preservative and sodium like regular canned soups. Of course, making your own is always best. See the recipe section for some good suggestion.

Q : WHAT DOES ORGANIC FOOD MEAN?

Organic foods are only those produced:
1. Without radiation
2. Without the use of conventional chemicals
3. Without the use of irradiation
4. Without bioengineering

Only foods that meet this criterion can be classified as certified organic and receive the "USDA Organic" seal.

Organic animal products must come from animals that have not been fed antibiotics and/or growth hormone and were fed an organic diet. Growers and producers must pass an inspection to be allowed to use the new label on their products.

The USDA has designated four categories of organic products:

1. 100% organic – must contain 100% organically produced ingredients
2. Organic – must contain at least 95% organic ingredients
3. Made with organic ingredients – must contain at least 70% organic ingredients
4. Some organic ingredients – may contain less than 70% organic ingredients

I recommend that you read the labels before purchasing food. 100% organic foods are richer in nutrients and free of pesticides and toxins.

Q : WHAT DOES A PH BALANCE MEAN?

Your PH balance is a measure of how acidic, or alkaline your body chemistry is. The human body is naturally slightly acidic. Ideally it should be 7.35 to 7.45, which is close to the neutral ph of 7.0 and is slightly alkaline. An excessive acidic diet of meat, sugar, and junk food causes the body to be more acidic which is the breeding ground for disease, especially cancer that thrives in a dark oxygen-starved acidic environment.

You can often see and smell over acidity as the body will excrete acid through the skin, developing acne, eczema, swelling, boils, eruptions, irritations, inflammations and general aches and pains. Your teeth may become sensitive to citrus and your urine may burn and smell acidic. Your stools may be hard, dry and foul smelling.

The main cause of over acidity is poor diet. Stress, emotional upheaval, and outside toxicity are contributing factors. The following are examples of acid and alkaline foods:

Acid- forming – tobacco, aspirin, most drugs, animal products such as meat, dairy, eggs and milk, processed and refined foods, yeast products, fermented foods, coffee, chocolate, sugar, alcohol, soft drinks and artificial sweeteners.

Alkaline-forming - most fruits and vegetables, sprouted seeds, nuts, avocadoes, corn, raisins, maple syrup, apricots, dates, grapefruit, grapes, honey, lemons, melons, molasses, oranges, figs and soy products.

Experts suggest you follow the 80%- 20% rule. Your acid forming part of your meal should be 20% and your alkaline forming foods should be 80%

You can perform a test at home to determine if your body is too acidic or alkaline. Purchase nitrazine – litmus paper at a drug store and apply saliva, or urine to the paper. Always perform the test before eating, or at least one hour after eating. Red litmus will turn blue in an alkaline state and blue litmus turns red in an acid state. Water is neutral at 7.0 so drink plenty of water.

Q : WHAT ARE ANTIOXIDANT AND FREE RADICALS?

We hear a lot about getting antioxidants into our diets, but few people understand why.

Antioxidants are a group of vitamins, minerals and enzymes that protect the body from the formation of free radicals. Your body keeps these free radicals in check by the use of free radical scavengers. These scavengers are certain enzymes that the body produces. However, they must be supplemented by the diet. We need to get plenty of vitamin A, E, C and the mineral selenium.

By definition a free radical is a chemical substance that contains an odd number of electrons. Every atom (chemical substance or mass) contains a certain number of electrons that orbit a nucleus- much like the solar system. Free radicals are made in the body all the time and if not destroyed can lead to cancer and other diseases. When high energy substances such as smoke, pollution, toxins, light, alcohol, stress, and polyunsaturated fats hit an atom, the energy kicks an electron out of balance, or orbit and transfers that energy to the electron which goes into a wild dance and is called a free radical.

The free radical is unstable and must get rid of the excess energy in order to stabilize. Hence the free radical seeks to transfer the energy to a near by substance (a healthy cell). All these reactions take place within a fraction of a second. When free radicals are made within the body, the high energy is transferred to body tissue, particularly to the polyunsaturated fats found in the cell membranes. The more polyunsaturated fats you eat, the higher the risk of membrane disruption because fat cells cannot fight the radical's attack.

Superoxide Dismutase, or SOD is an enzyme that neutralizes free radicals. It is assisted by the antioxidants A, E, and C. A healthy body produces about 5 million units of the enzyme SOD. SOD revitalizes the cells and reduces the rate of cell destruction. It removes the most common free radical, superoxide. SOD also aids the body's utilization of zinc, copper and manganese. With aging free radical production increases, while SOD levels are reduced. SOD naturally occurs in foods such as barley, broccoli, cabbage, Brussel sprouts, and wheat grass. All these foods are high in vitamin A.

Vitamin E is a powerful antioxidant. It is important that it be tocopherol and tocotrienol; the chemical properties that make E, truly vitamin E. A study from the researchers at the Antioxidant Research Laboratory at Tuft's University in Boston suggest that vitamin E may help to alleviate muscle soreness caused by free radicals that are by products of oxygen metabolism, which can damage and cause fatigue to muscle tissues after a workout.

There is a measure of antioxidants called the ORAC scale – (oxygen radical antioxidant capacity), which is a measure of the antioxidant capacity found in foods. The top of the scale rates prunes, spinach, strawberries and blueberries as foods highest in antioxidants. Researchers suggest that a diet rich in spinach and blueberries may help prevent age related mental declines such as Alzheimer's and Parkinson's disease. Studies suggest that life long accumulation of free radicals in the brain may be linked to age related mental decline. To date the study has only been conducted on rats and should now be tested on humans.

Q : SHOULD I EAT CARBOHYDRATES AND OR PROTEIN BEFORE OR AFTER I WORK OUT?

New data suggest that it is important to get both carbohydrates and protein after a workout. Suggested is that you eat a light complex carbohydrate meal just before the workout for immediate fuel and energy, and then within an hour after the workout combine carbohydrates with protein for rebuilding and refueling power.

The suggestion is that you get 2-4 grams of carbohydrates to 1 gram of protein, post workout. The jury is still out on how long and how much, however a good rule of thumb would be to eat some complex carbohydrates and some lean protein within an hour or two of your workouts.

It is important to maintain lean muscle mass while burning fat. People who exercise are at risk of chromium deficiencies because chromium is involved in the metabolism of glucose, which is the fuel, needed for energy. Chromium is vital in the synthesis of cholesterol, fat and protein. This mineral stabilizes blood sugar levels through proper insulin utilization. Zinc is another mineral that is lost through strenuous exercise due to increased glucose metabolism. Complex carbohydrates and lean proteins supply the fuel to workout and to rebuild.

Q : HERBS AND SPICES –
HOW DO THEY FIT INTO A HEALTHY DIET?

When we think of herbs we think of medicinal plants and when we think of spices we think of seasonings. Actually, spices and herbs are both plants, and the line between the two is somewhat blurred. There are herbs that are used medically that you would not use to season your foods, and most spices are not what we would use for herbal medicine. Since this is a book on food, this question will pertain mostly to spices and culinary herbs. But first let me briefly mention some important medicinal herbs.

I created a nectar for the immune system using medicinal herbs. It's called Pep Berry Rob, after an old remedy called a rob which used elderberries as its many ingredients. My nectar combines elderberries, with Echinacea, astragalas, rose hips, ginseng, sarsaparilla and licorice; all herbs that are known to boost the immune system through their content of important vitamins and minerals. This nectar in a base of honey and natural flavoring to boost the immune system, giving you the energy and the help to protect against colds and flues. For more information go to www.doctorlynn.com

The most common culinary herbs and spices are often added to foods for flavor; however, they also offer medicinal properties and might have been originally added to foods for that purpose.

Most culinary herbs and spices aid digestion and relieve nervousness. Thus, the kitchen spice rack may be thought of as a small natural pharmacy. Let's look at some of the better-known herbs and spices.
Basil – in Italy the fragrant basil is given to a loved one as a pledge of fidelity and young men wear a sprig behind their ear when they go courting. Basil is a very fragrant herb that is a tonic, stimulant and

calmative. It is used to improve appetite, relieve fatigue, and heal intestinal problems.

Bay leaf – the bay tree was considered capable of increasing and maintaining health and happiness. One or two bay leaves added to a soup or beans improve the flavor and helps prevent gas and indigestion.

Black Pepper – black pepper is an excellent remedy at the first sign of disease. Yogis consider black pepper to be one of nature's most perfect foods and useful as a preventative food. According to expert's black pepper contains four anti-osteoporosis compounds. Therefore, it might be wise to use it generously on your foods. Yogis mix seven ground peppercorns (one-eighth teaspoon of powder) with a tablespoon of honey each morning. The mixture is said to overcome mucus and sore throats.

Caraway - caraway is excellent for digestion. It is taken for indigestion, gas, colic and nervous conditions. Just steep a few seeds in a cup of boiling water and drink.

Cardamom – is a calmative usually mixed with other spices to treat indigestion. It is an important Indian spice used in many dishes.

Cayenne – the genus Capsicum includes red and green chilies, cayenne, paprika and bell peppers. Cayenne is a stimulant, taken daily to benefit the heart and circulation. Cayenne is a hot spice that will add a lot of flavor and flare to your foods as well as useful as a medicinal spice. Use it internally to improve circulation and externally to reduce inflammation. If you combined it with a plantain and apply as a poultice it will draw out foreign objects embedded in the flesh. Cayenne and paprika are also good sources of potassium.

Cinnamon - is a warm and inviting spice. It is used by the Chinese to increase circulation and produce warming. It is used to bring balance to cold foods such as fruits, milk and desserts. Simmered in milk and taken with honey it is great for indigestion.

Cloves like cinnamon and allspice are warming and stimulating to the body. They improve circulation and improve digestion. Oil of clove gives quick relief to toothaches and cloves may be chewed for this purpose.

Cumin - cumin is an essential ingredient in making curries. It is one of the best spices to use in preventing and relieving gas. Cumin has three pain-relieving compounds, seven anti-inflammatory and four that combat swelling. It is sometimes used to relieve carpel tunnel syndrome. Eat lots of cumin and add it to curried rice.

Garlic – considered one of the most important medicinal foods, is world renowned as a cure-all in practically every culture. The ingredient that gives garlic its strong smell, a chemical called allicin, is also what makes it such a potent antibiotic. In hundreds of experiments, allicin extract from raw garlic has destroyed the germs that spread such diseases as botulism, tuberculosis, diarrhea, staph, dysentery and typhoid.

Like chili peppers and other hot pungent foods, garlic works to turn on the body's natural fighting element to cool the heat. This provokes the lungs and bronchial tubes to produce more fluids, which thins mucus, helping to flush it out of the body.

Cooking may destroy some of the allicin, but most of its therapeutic benefits remain. Garlic lowers blood cholesterols, is a cancer fighter, blocks germs, is an anti- microbe fighter and a significant antibiotic, as well as a decongestant.

Whether cooked or raw, garlic may be one of the most potent natural healing foods. Before the birth of Christ, the Israelis were using garlic as a major ingredient in their foods, as well as a medicine.

Ginger – is one of the most versatile herbal stimulants. It is used for the stomach, intestines and for circulation. It is one of the best remedies for nausea. Grating fresh ginger and letting it steep in hot water makes a great ginger tea. Add a little honey and lemon, and it is a great cold remedy. Ginger root, it is recommended should be added to meat dishes to help your intestines detoxify the meat. Ginger root is eaten with sushi to aid digestion. Squeeze out the juice of fresh ginger and add it to equal parts of olive oil and sesame oil and use it as a rub for the relief of muscle pain. It is best to always use fresh ginger, but dried may also be used.

Marjoram – is a carminative tonic herb used for upset stomach. It is considered helpful for seasickness. The oil of marjoram is applied externally to relieve pain. When added to a bath it has a calming effect and relieves insomnia. It is a fragrant herb used like oregano, bay and sage in stews, soups, meat dishes and egg and cheese dishes.

Mustard Seeds - ancient wisdom tells us that mustard seeds are for good luck. Internally the crushed seed acts as a mild laxative and blood purifier. Externally mustard can be applied as a plaster and used to relieve aches and pains.

Nutmeg – a small amount of nutmeg can be used daily to relieve chronic nervous disorders and heart problems. It may be added to milk and baked fruits and desserts to help digestion and relieve nausea. Large dosages can be poisonous and may cause miscarriage.

Rosemary – is used to treat headaches, as well as used for insomnia. It is rich in easily assimilated calcium and thus good for the entire nervous system. It is useful for indigestion, gas and fevers.

Sage - the planet Jupiter, the benevolent planet that supports good nutrition and health, governs Sage. There an expression that describes the ancient value of sage in the garden; "He who has sage in his garden has nothing to fear." The active ingredient in sage is a volatile oil. It is a stimulant, astringent, tonic, calmative and disinfectant. Sage is wonderfully fragrant herb that has many wonderful uses. Sprinkle fresh sage on warm vegetables, or on top of scrambled eggs, or omelets. It is used in stuffing not only for its flavor, but to prevent against indigestion. Rub sage and sea salt together as a homemade teeth-whitening agent.

Thyme – As a healthy culinary herb, thyme enhances the flavor of soups, stuffing and homemade mayonnaise. It makes a fragrant herb flavor sprinkled on beets, carrots, or parsnips. Thyme is an antiseptic and calmative herb used to treat colds and fungus infections. It is safe and effective as a tea for indigestion. Its fragrance attracts bees and gives a delightful flavor to honey.

Turmeric – East Indians use turmeric quite liberally in their curries. Aside from adding a lot of flavor turmeric is known for its ability to stimulate the adrenal glands by releasing a chemical compound called curcumin, which is a pain reliever. It has also been used to relieve the pain of ulcers. In an Asian study 250-milligrams of turmeric capsules were taken three times per day to relieve ulcer pain. Turmeric is an antioxidant herb.

Lab test have determined that herbs such as cinnamon, nutmeg, cumin, garlic, clove, onion and celery neutralize food borne microbes such as E.coli. Sprinkle these spices on your foods and add celery, onion and garlic to your diet.

There are numerous herbs and spices that will add both flavor and health to your meals. Try adding parsley and cilantro for flavor and to clean the palette. Remember this expression, "variety is the spice of life." We should use a variety of taste and nutrients to keep our health in balance. Spices and herbs can help to keep your digestive fires burning properly. This is one of the ways to maintain metabolism and maintain your ideal weight. The best way to ensure you are getting enough of the taste that will balance your energy is to add a variety of spices and herbs to your life. Herbs and spices add taste without adding calories.

THE YOGI DIET

U sing foods to bring body-mind balance into our lives takes self-discipline, patience and commitment to your health. It is the difference between practicing a lifestyle of prevention and suffering the consequences of trying to cure a disease, or malady. Anna-maya-kosha-yoga teaches us to take responsibility for our health and well being. Along with practicing yoga and daily forms of exercise we need to develop a positive mental attitude, which can be achieved through meditation and sleep. Exercise and peaceful restful sleep are considered two of the three great pillars of health and balance. The third great pillar is the foods we eat.

Modern scientific research has confirmed that we can enhance our health and, in some cases, prevent disease, through good nutrition. When we do not give the body proper nutrition, we risk doing great harm to our selves by impairing the body's normal functions. The problem for most of us is through our modern-day diet we may not be getting the proper nutrients. Even if we are not sick, we may not in fact be healthy. It may simply be that we are not exhibiting any overt symptoms. By practicing the principles of Anna-maya-kosha-yoga, which is holistic nutrition, we can improve the state of our health, perhaps stave off disease, and maintain a harmonious balance, just as nature intended.

Before we can begin to eat the yogi way, we need to detoxify the system. The following detoxification program is a simple cleanse to get rid of toxins.

FASTING - DETOXIFICATION

F asting means more than just not eating. There is both a science and an art to the process of fasting. When we think of fasting, we think of abstention from all food. We often equate this with starvation; however, fasting and starvation are not the same. The former is life sustaining and the latter is life harming.

In religious terms fasting means the total abstinence from certain foods on Holy days. This is what we call a "partial" abstinence, because often times, as in Lent, one food is substituted for another. Anna-maya-kosha yoga in its strictest sense promotes eating little and fasting often. However, we should keep in mind that the ancient philosophies of yoga were written in ancient times, for another culture and applicable to another lifestyle. Modern day lifestyles and western cultures are not necessarily conducive to a strict fast.

Keep in mind that the basic foundation of Anna-maya-kosha-yoga is to do no harm. Further it is abstaining from those things (foods) that bring us harm that is the conscious path of Anna-maya-kosha-yoga.

For centuries humans all over the world have employed fasting for religious reasons, political reasons, for self-discipline, and as a means of restoring health. The Bible, Homer, and even Hippocrates made use of fasting to care for the sick. Animals of all kinds use fasting as a method of curing disease. Nature herself uses pain, fever, gastric congestion, and even mental afflictions to take away appetite. It is only in the last century that we have been taught to eat to keep up our strength. The critics of fasting are usually those who have never missed a meal in their lives!

Fasting again does not mean going without food. Its literal translation comes from the English word *faesten*, which means firm or fixed. It is something that we hold onto under fixed and controlled conditions. For our purposes we are going to focus on detoxification by using a controlled and fixed eating plan. Detoxification is simply a cleansing method to remove toxic energy from the body-mind.

A gentle internal cleansing will help to clear the body of lactic acid, toxic gas, waste, and phylum, or mucus. A detoxification program allows the digestive system to take a break by only eating soft liquid foods. Solid foods require many hours of digestive activity before its nutritional value is available to the cells and tissues of the body.

The purpose of a detoxification program is not to lose weight, although you may lose weight by first applying the program and then adhering to a weight reduction program. The primary goal is to rid the body-mind of toxic build up, waste, lactic acid, and phlegm and mucus.

In nature the automatic balance is the delicate contrast between expansion and contraction. This is what brings all things into balance. Nature must expand in one area and likewise will contract in another. So, if food is taken into the body to be digested (expand) much blood must flow to the digestive organs and we tend to become sluggish and sleepy (contract).

Partial fasting (detoxification) conserves the energy used for digestion and converts it to other parts of the body. In other words, we contract our digestion and expand our energy. In a general sense the more food one eats the more work must be performed by the digestive and elimination organs. With a reduction in food, these organs rest. When organs, or for that matter any part of the body is at rest it has an opportunity to rebuild and rejuvenate the cellular structure of the body. As the glands and organs slow done the respiration slows and the nervous system has less work to do. The body-mind slows and begins to build and find its balance.

Detoxification will purify the blood and remove toxic waste from the body. It increases the elimination of waste from the blood and tissues. As pent-up waste is removed the body more effectively and efficiently uses nutrition to restore the organism. Excretion of waste and toxins is a fundamental function of maintaining proper health. To maintain health the body-mind must employ the laws of balance, whereby on one hand it employs assimilation and growth, and on the other hand it employs excretion and the removal of waste.

There is a theory that the body cannot excrete waste while it is busy digesting. This is not completely true, as excretion must go on even while food is being digested, or we would build up toxic waste resulting in self poisoning. Therefore, it is safer to suspend digestion for a brief time rather than suspend excretion. This is why Anna-maya-kosha-yoga states that we should eat little and fast regularly. Over consumption of foods and especially foods of little nutritional value compromise a healthy and balanced body-mind.

Waste and toxins are stored in the body tissues, especially in the fatty and connective tissues, and as these tissues are liquefied through the detoxification process the toxin are released. Without proper elimination, toxins and waste caught in the tissues and fecal matter become lodged in the intestines and are subject to the same flow of blood that makes it way to the brain. Therefore, a sluggish digestive system also causes a sluggish mental system.

Through the detoxification process the body mobilizes all its reserves including deposited waste products, and through the process of oxidation (oxygen) eliminates them from the system. The symptoms of bloating, gas, skin irritations, sinus congestion, indigestion, headaches, body aches, agitation, sluggishness and depression are eradicated. The excretion removes toxic waste and restores the body-mind system, removing the systems of toxicity and restoring the body to a state of balance.

Remember: Anna-maya-kosha-yoga reminds us to do no harm, and to seek balance in all things, and in all things find balance.

By now you are aware of the foods, herbs, and spices that will help to maximize your digestion. You should now be more aware of the fats, proteins and carbohydrates that will keep you in balance.

Before beginning any kind of a fasting/detoxification program you should check with your general practitioner. Various health conditions and medication may prevent you from doing such an extensive program. The following detoxification program should be safe for most anyone as it is not a strict fast, but a program to safely eliminate toxic energy from the system.

As in all human activities, wisdom and common sense should prevail. In most cases the detoxification program under proper guidance and for the proper duration should leave the individual stronger in both physical and mental capacities.

The following detoxification program is a three-day program whereby we eat a pure and whole diet for the first day and the third day. The second day we use the detoxification diet. It is perfectly safe to use the detoxification day for two/three days in a row. However, in a modern-day western world it is somewhat difficult to take the time away from family, activities, and work to indulges self with relaxation and purification of the body-mind. The day of detoxification should be a day when you have no activities such as exercise, or work. It is a time for quietude, relaxation and reflection. This is the time to honor you. It is not a deprivation, but a health-giving gift to you. Make this a special day for yourself by honoring that which gives you health.

THE PROGRAM

The purpose of the three-day detoxification program is to rid the body of caffeine, wheat, gluten, sugar, simple carbohydrates, fats, meats and other denatured foods. We are not trying to lose weight, but rather to bring radiant health to the body-mind.

The program will start with a day of eating whole live foods, followed by a day of detoxification and then a day of whole live foods. Whole live foods mean, foods that are not cooked or processed. This would be fruits, vegetables, juices, soy powder or tofu, cottage cheese, goat's cheeses, nuts, peanut butter, natural whole grains. Meat, cooked foods, and processed foods are to be eliminated.

The following is a grocery list of foods and products
you will need to have on hand.

1. Fresh lemons
2. Honey
3. Fresh Ginger
4. Fresh fruits; bananas, melons, apples, pears, berries
5. Aloe Vera Juice
6. Organic apple juice, cranberry juice or grape juice 4 ounces = 1 serving
7. Organic carrot, beet, celery juice or combination of carrot juice with any other vegetable. 16 ounces = 1 serving
8. Green tea and assorted herbal teas

9. Kefir – plain organic 32 oz - a liquid yogurt product (may also use plain organic yogurt

10. Cinnamon, curry powder, turmeric

11. Protein powder – soy and whey or just soy, whey or rice – 1 can – 12 oz

12. Liquid milk thistle tincture – can be found in a health food store

13. Organic vegetable broth – can be bought in a health food store

14. Vegetables - onions, mushrooms, kale, broccoli, cabbage, spinach, carrots

15. Lettuce – tomatoes

16. Tofu - cottage cheese – goats' cheese

17. Pure peanut butter with no additives

18. Nuts – almonds, walnuts

19. Whole grain – organic bread

• All foods are optional – you may eat all of the foods included in the next three days plan or any portion thereof, but do not eat outside the following foods. This is not a diet, but a detoxification program so it is important to eat only the foods listed in the program.

DAY 1 - WHOLE FOOD DIET

Morning
- Green tea with honey and ginger or herbal tea
- Organic juice – 4 oz.
- 1 Slice whole grain bread with peanut butter or cottage cheese
- Fruit – sliced banana or melon with 1 tablespoon kefir

Mid Morning
- Apple or pear

Lunch
- Salad of greens, tomatoes, 1/2 cottage cheese, soy cheese or goat cheese
- 1 slice of whole grain bread with peanut butter or honey
- Sliced fruit – melon, banana, apple, grapes – your preference

Mid afternoon
- Apple or any fruit mixed with a banana and 3 oz of kefir
- A serving of soy/whey powder and
- 2 ounces of water – mix in blender and drink.
  Try freezing the banana in its peel. Run the banana under hot water, peel, and cut into chunks and use in the shake. This will make it thicker and more like a smoothie.

Evening meal
- A large salad of greens, tomatoes, chopped raw vegetables, olive oil and balsamic dressing with tofu, cottage cheese or goat cheese * see recipes - roasted beet, onion and goat cheese salad for dinner suggestion
- Slice of whole grain bread with peanut butter or honey
- Fresh sliced fruit plate

• Herbal tea with or without honey and ginger -

Nothing to eat after 7:00 PM accept, herbal tea with honey and ginger in the evening.

DAY 2 - DETOXIFICATION

Morning
• Green tea with honey and ginger or herbal tea with honey and ginger
• 4 oz of organic apple, cranberry or grape juice mixed with 1 tablespoon of aloe Vera juice and
• *1 dropper full of milk thistle optional

Nine AM or mid morning
Protein shake – the purpose of the shake is to keep the blood sugar level and to support the liver so that it can perform its function of detoxifying.
• 2 scoops of soy/whey protein or whey protein or rice protein
• 3 ounces of warm water
• 3 ounces of kefir
• 1 banana - frozen
• 3 or 4 fresh berries
• ¼ teaspoon of cinnamon

Blend together and drink. Through the rest of the morning drink herbal tea, lemon and honey

Noon
Repeat protein shake

Afternoon
- Fresh organic vegetable juice – 16 ounces

Continue to drink herbal teas with honey and lemon

4 PM – or late afternoon

Repeat protein shake

6 PM – or evening meal not later than 7:00 PM
- Sauté vegetable mixture – (your choice) in a little olive oil and add to vegetable broth. Heat until the vegetables are soft. It is not necessary to puree, just eat the broth and vegetables. If you would like add a little curry and turmeric for taste or any other spice you like such as black pepper or oregano.

Evening
- Have herbal tea with a little honey and lemon.
- Add a dropper full of milk thistle. (optional)

DAY 3 - REPEAT DAY 1

Now start on day 4 eating a healthy diet of whole foods combined with whole grains (complex carbohydrates) and add fish, eggs, chicken, good fats and other healthy foods into your diet. Continue to take the milk thistle once a day in your juice for the next two weeks, ***optional for liver cleansing.** Try to stay with the green tea and give up the coffee.

After cleanse you should be feeling a bit lighter, brighter and calmer. Remember it is not about losing weight, but about removing toxic energy from your body-mind. Using this detoxification program will also help to jump-start you into eating the yoga way of Anna-maya-kosha.

If your diet has been really heavy with denatured foods, junk foods and processed foods it may take a bit of patience. If you find that you cannot stick with the three-day plan, don't get discouraged. Take the time to reflect upon what it is that is blocking you from giving up that which is doing you harm and embracing that which gives you healthy sustaining life.

This detoxification program is perfectly safe to do four times a year or at the beginning of each season. Always check with your primary caregiver before embarking upon any detoxification program, diet program or new exercise program.

Contrary to some professional opinions, the vital tissues of the body do not waste away during a detoxification, or fasting program. The fasting body will lose weight, but it is not of the tissues, but of the reserves of fat and toxins. In periods of abstinence, it is fat cells that are lost and not muscle tissue. Weight loss is determined by character and quality of the tissues of the individual, the amount of physical and emotional activity, and temperature surrounding the body. Physical activity, emotional stress and cold and poor tissues all provide for faster weight loss. However, this is not always the best for the body-mind. We are striving for balance and balance means we find peace and calmness in the body-mind.

Remember the Buddha said that once we reach a state of soulful awareness, we cannot help but live a healthy life. Aware of our journey we seek only that which honors the body-mind for the body-mind is the vehicle of the soul. Your journey is about the discovery of wisdom and that is achieved, according to yoga, through the long learning process of life. Healthy choices support the long learning process of life.

As we become more and more aware of our soulful strength, our physical and mental self becomes a reflection of this awareness. From the power of the soul an inner strength emerges, providing the awareness of choice. Choice allows us the opportunity to make decisions, and solve problems in such a way as to reflect the true nature of our self. Our true nature is a unifying force where the boundaries of ego and the struggle for power give way to balance and peace. This is the center of empowerment.

This center of empowerment known as the third charka, is the seat of the individualized consciousness or the ego. It is the store house of prana, which is the force that gives life to the universe. Because it is located in the gut area, it is related to digestion and the absorption of food. When malfunctioning its related diseases are diabetes, obesity, ulcers, and gall bladder, and liver problems.

When we harness this soulful energy, making lifestyle changes becomes an easy choice. But how do we harness this energy? It begins with a desire to get healthy. Anything can be achieved, once we harness the eternal soulful energy of desire. This inner desire is the fuel that supports all creation. To be mentally and physically healthy is to support desire with the inner strength of the soul. This inner strength brings changes that are lasting and enduring because we are correcting the energy of imbalances on all levels. There cannot be a correction in one area without the others, if true healing (health) is to occur.

This is why diets and exercise programs don't work. We only attempt to correct the problem by focusing on the physical level. We neglect the emotional aspect of health, and forget that it is from the soulful energy that all things manifest. Affirmations of the mind don't work because they are only tied to one layer of energy. When we create (see ourselves in health) from the soulful realm, the physical and mental world reflects this manifestation.

This is the key to the mastery of life. Any obstacle can be overcome and transformed into a strength that will endure, provided we get healthy and balanced on all levels, body, mind, and soul. When you choose from the level of your soul to correct the energy of the body-mind you empower yourself with the eternal strength of will power. In Anna-maya-kosha yoga we focus on health and not on dieting through the soulful power of free will.

With Anna-maya-kosha-yoga sticking to a healthy eating plan, an exercise program, and daily soulful practice will become natural, instinctual, and blissful. Motivation simply becomes a state of being, and from this state of being, comes a lifestyle of health, grace, and nobility.

If you are reading this, you may be searching for something, curious about alternatives, or in the middle of a crisis. All three present you with an opportunity to grow. This program is not a diet program, but rather a look at simple lifestyle changes that can bring dramatic changes to your life. The most important aspect is to learn to love you. This is not a selfish love, but rather an appreciation for the uniqueness of you. Take a moment and look around you. You will see all sorts of people in various shapes and sizes. All have a quality of beauty, and all are important. The ones that shine through with the greatest beauty are the ones that have learned to take their own importance and use it to serve others.

No matter what your station in life, true fulfillment comes not from self-gratification, but from serving humanity.

More importantly don't get caught up in the media illusion of the perfect body. True beauty is about health in body, mind, and soul. Having a healthy self image combined with a healthy lifestyle of diet and exercise creates enduring beauty.

During the three-day cleanse you should not do any high-energy activities. This is a time of relaxation and reflection. Use it as a time to read, meditate, take a hot aromatherapy bath, rest and enjoy a bit of quietude.

In quietude we learn to quiet the mind, speak few words, and act with balance. When this is accomplished, all that we think, say, and do will be beautiful and meaningful

EAT LIKE A YOGI

F oods in their natural (preferably organic state) provide the proteins, carbohydrates, fats, vitamins and minerals that the body-mind needs to achieve health and balance. The vegetarian diet does supply essential nutrients while maintaining a purity of body-mind.

The ancient practice of eating like a yogi was to eliminate meat and eggs from the diet and to limit the intake of dairy products except for organic yogurt, milk and soy. This was known as the practice of *ahimsa*, the Sanskrit word for non-violence towards animals and in a larger sense towards the planetary environment.

I believe most would agree that eating less or no meat is a healthy choice, however our Western culture and lifestyles need to be considered. Yoga teaches us to do no harm and that means not to harm self. The laws of karma teach us that every cause (action) has an effect. Events (food choices) are not to be looked upon as bad or good, but rather symbols of our attitudes towards ourselves and our world.

It is important to remember that which causes a soul to expand is good karma and that which causes a soul to contract is bad karma, however what cause one soul to expand or contract is not necessarily true for another soul. The most important thing you can do to override karma is to be consistent. What you want today may differ from what you wanted yesterday and yet you must live today with the desires of yesterday, so be sure what you want today is what you will want tomorrow. In other words, make sure the junk food you want today will be what you want tomorrow for it will be in your life in terms of weight gain and lethargic feelings tomorrow. The yogi diet teaches that we should always choose that which brings the greatest good and leads to the greatest happiness.

On a subtle level the science of yoga teaches that food is nourishing in proportion to the amount of prana life energy that it embodies. Fresh, whole foods prepared with mindful awareness, contain the maximum amount of health-giving energy. In India the master chef is both a cook and a holistic healer, feeding body, mind and soul.

The food plan and the recipes are made from ingredients that are believed to provide health-giving properties in and of themselves. Equally important is the positive attitudes and love with which they are prepared and served. Singing, smiling and consciously relaxing while preparing and serving a meal infuses the food with vitality and peace-giving properties. Taking a few moments to give thanks for the meal, then eating in appreciation, while slowly savoring each bite, produces maximum soulful, mental and physical nourishment.

Most of the foods included in this book are based upon the yogic way of eating adapted to a western lifestyle. The traditional yogic diet is lacto-vegetarianism (fruits, vegetables, grains, yogurt and milk). This plan includes these foods but expands upon the basics using spices and western foods to develop a diet that is focused more on health and balance than any hard and fast ideology. It is important to remember that it is not about following a prescribed way of life to the letter. The yogic path is that of the individual striving to find inner peace and balance.

THE PLAN

N ow that we understand the principles of Anna-maya-kosha-yoga, which is eating with a purpose, it's time to get started. Changing your way of eating may at first seems a bit overwhelming, but with a little self discipline and a desire to bring health to your body-mind, the process will be made a lot easier.

First, I'll give you some basic guidelines that you can adapt so as to create delicious, quick, and wholesome meals for yourself and your family. Remember Anna-maya-kosha-yoga is about a lifestyle and not about losing weight. It is about the choices we make to honor the body-mind through good nutrition.

As already discussed, eating and cooking fresh whole foods, herbs, and spices is really much easier and faster than eating the processed foods that you have been used to eating. First you need to clean your cupboard of all the unhealthy foods and begin to fill the refrigerator and cupboard with health giving foods.

Choose fresh ingredients and whole foods. The fresher the food the closer they are to their natural state and the more flavor they will have without a lot of additives. Simply adding spices and herbs and keeping foods in their natural state create delicious meals.

Most of the foods that Americans eat are recipes that were brought over by the early European settlers. However, modern-day life has adapted most of these foods to a society of fast and immediate meals.

Most foods are processed for efficiency. Forty-seven percent of American meals are take-out or eaten in a restaurant. Many of the old traditional recipes are disappearing as Americans cook less and less, and rely more on ready to eat and processed foods. The secret is to make a conscious choice to buy and prepare whole flavorful and healthy foods in the home, and when dining out make healthy food choices. Use lots of herbs and spices to add flavor, health and excitement to your food.

Two diets that are promoted as being healthy are the Mediterranean diet and the Asian diet. If you look at both of these diets, very little meat is consumed with a lot of fish, vegetables, fruits and whole grains being the staple of the diets. Sweets and alcohol are limited.

If you follow the basic food laws of 6 servings of vegetables per day, two - four servings of fruit per day, the proper amount of protein per day (grams to weight according to your level of exercise), eliminate dairy except for yogurt and kefir, and limit your carbohydrates to complex carbohydrates, which include whole grains, you will be getting a healthy diet.

When you eat a diet that is balanced in complex carbohydrates, lean proteins, and good fats you will achieve a ratio of 20% acid foods to 80% alkaline foods. This ratio supports a healthy internal environment. An easy way to achieve this is to eat one grain with several vegetables at one meal, and one protein with several vegetables at another meal. Eat fruit in between meals. Of course, you should only use this as a rule of thumb. Use the information in this book to design your eating plan according to your lifestyle. If you exercise a lot, you need more carbohydrates and more proteins.

Weight gains are often as a result of eating too many carbohydrates and a low protein diet. A low protein diet will lead to low blood sugar levels that in turn will, lead to hunger and cravings for carbohydrates. When blood sugar levels drop, we tend to reach for quick simple sugary carbohydrates. That is why I designed the detoxification plan using the protein shakes to keep the blood sugar levels even.

Another factor is the neurotransmitter serotonin, which is a precursor to the amino acid tryptophan. Tryptophan is the feel-good neurotransmitter and is the chemical in our brain that is responsible for satiety. Too much protein can inhibit the uptake of tryptophan. Complex carbohydrates such as stabilized rice bran provide tryptophan. We need to balance out both the protein and complex carbohydrates to keep the body-mind in a place of healthy consciousness.

To manage your weight and/or to lose weight you might want to add a couple of things to your diet. Researchers have found that red pepper and other hot spices, as well as mustard and horse radish or wasabi (sushi) raised metabolic rates by 25 percent. Spicy foods also stimulate thirst, so you drink more water, and the more water you drink the fuller you get without adding calories.

Another food to add to the diet is pineapple. Pineapple contains the enzyme bromelain, which helps the digestion of proteins and fats. Pineapple is also high in vitamin C, and is an alkaline food.

The journey to a healthy balanced diet is up to you. Remember every journey begins with the first step. Here are some strategies for changing your diet. If you follow this plan within thirty days you will change your entire eating habits.

1. Clean out your cupboards and refrigerator. Start now and throw out all fat-free and sugar free foods. Throw out anything containing sugar or high fructose corn syrup. Rid your food pantry of all white flours and simple carbohydrates. Remove white rice, pastas, white bread, and sugar. Eliminate all starchy vegetables such as potatoes and corn. Throw out all soft drinks, sugary fruit juices and alcohol (accept may-be red wine). Remember alcohol should only be consumed in moderation, as it is high in simple sugars. Throw out all your cooking oils and start cooking with cold pressed, extra virgin olive oil.

2. Now fill your cupboards with complex carbohydrates (whole grains), fresh vegetables, and fruits, and plenty of lean protein. Oat meal, rice bran, soy products, legumes, fresh vegetables and fruits provide lots of good fiber and will fill you up while providing nutrients to the body-mind.

3. At every meal try to eat a little protein. Protein stimulates the production of glucagons, the hormone that counters insulin and helps your body burn stored fats and carbohydrates. Make smart protein choices such as lean chicken and turkey, fish and seafood, eggs and soy products. Eliminate all processed meats and heavy fatty meats.

4. Exercises prevent the build up of body fat and help the digestive system to more effectively and efficiently use its fuel. Try to find 20 to 30 minutes a day to take a walk or do yoga stretches. Not only will you burn calories, but you will also produce endorphins in the brain and these feel-good neurochemicals help us to stop the cravings and feel a sense of relaxation.

The body changes according to what we feed it. It will mold towards salads and fresh healthy foods, or it can be molded towards junk foods. Your body does the best it can with what foods you eat. When you change your diet to a proper healthy balanced way of eating your whole body-mind changes with it.

Here is a typical eating plan for a day:

Morning – green tea with honey, stevia (an all-natural non-caloric sweetener that can be found in health food stores) or plain. Drink 4 oz of fresh organic fruit juice. A complex carbohydrate such as a serving of oatmeal or whole grain granola or cereal with a couple of tablespoons of kefir, nuts for protein and ¼ chopped banana and a few berries. Or a slice of whole grain toast with a tablespoon of peanut butter and sliced banana and melons.

Mid – morning – a piece of fruit such as an apple

Lunch – steamed vegetables, a garden salad and a lean piece of fish, chicken or a serving of soy, goat cheese or eggs. Fruit for dessert.

Mid – afternoon – a serving of fruit or a protein shake or an 8 oz glass of vegetable juice.

Dinner – steamed vegetables, whole grain serving such as brown rice, basmati rice, or any other whole grain complex carbohydrate. A 4-6 oz serving of fresh salt, or fresh water fish. Salmon, tuna, or halibut would be good choices. Or a 4-6 oz serving of chicken, or lean meat. Try to eat farm raised organic poultry and meats. Fruit for dessert, (try some of the healthy dessert recipes given in the next section.

Drink lots of water and herbal teas. Indulge occasionally in a piece of chocolate or a dessert. Choose dark organic chocolate and desserts that are fruit desserts and not heavy in creams and sauces.

This eating plan is not about losing weight, but about eating a healthy and balanced diet. If you eat whole foods and eliminate processed and rich foods from your diet you will notice that you can eat well, not feel hungry, and will have a lot more energy. Your weight will be maintained and your sleeping, playing and working energy will be enhanced. Eat as close to natural as possible and graze throughout the day. Never let the blood sugar dip to levels where you are ravenous and begin to reach for quick snacks with out consciously thinking about what you are eating. Anna-maya-kosha-yoga is about the consciousness of eating, for you are what and how you eat.

Use the following recipes as guideline for choices of foods to cook at home and for food to choose when eating out. The way of the yogi is the path that brings the greatest good, is harmonious, and brings balance and peace into your life. The greatest gift of life is life itself. To live a long and radiant life is said to have the great opportunity to gain wisdom which is the ultimate purpose of our existence.

Anna-maya-kosha-yoga is the path that follows the principle that eating healthy supports the temple of the soul (the body-mind) and this gives one the opportunity to experience the bliss and joy of life. The fundamental principles of Anna-maya-kosha-yoga are to inspect what and how you eat. Yoga is all-inclusive and no aspect of life should be ignored, including what and how you eat.

Dining Out

A bout 47 percent of our meals are eaten out in restaurants or through take –out. Busy Western lifestyles make it difficult to cook and eat home cooked meals. It seems sometimes that the most important thing in the modern restaurant is not the food but the concept. So, what is a yogi to do when faced with eating out? Well, if you are strict vegetarian than that limits you to vegetarian restaurants and/or restaurants that usually have a limited vegetarian menu.

Tips for eating out:

- Seek restaurants that serve organic foods. Read the menus and you might be surprised to see such things as free range or organic.
- Avoid white and beige colored foods. These foods are usually potatoes, breads and French fires. When ordering, think color. Green, red, orange and yellow foods usually are better choices.
- Don't fill up on bread. It's wasted calories.
- Order water with lemon. Lemon is a purifier and aids the digestive system.
- After dinner have hot herbal tea. Studies have shown that hot tea helps to metabolize fat in the diet.
- For dessert order fruit or sorbet.
- Share your meal with other. It's more interesting and we tend to eat less when we share our food.
- Eat slowly and chew your food. Be very Zen with your dining experience. When you're dining, simply eat and enjoy the food and the experience.

RESTAURANT WE'D LIKE TO SEE

With 18 million people doing yoga, you'd think we'd see a restaurant concept of the Anna-maya-kosha-yoga approach to eating. What about a yogi restaurant? Try to imagine this...

Soft candle lit rooms, with mystical peaceful music softly playing in the background. Once you enter the restaurant you step into the Zen moment of simply experiencing the joy of eating. You are escorted to a quiet table that is low to the ground. Cushions surround the table. You sit around the table on the cushions in easy pose (simple cross leg position).

The server appears, bows and in a soft and warm voice welcomes you. You are handed a menu that resemble fine parchment and hand inscribed. Inside the menus you see that the choices are divided according to the colors of the charkas (energy centers). The food choices are designed to support and enhance whichever charkas you wish to feed with healthy foods. Within each color would be foods especially designed for the charka energy.

The effects of color on our moods and health have been studied and documented by scientist. Red stimulates and excites the body. Orange stimulates appetite and reduces fatigue. Yellow stimulates memory and lifts spirits. Green is balancing, stimulates metabolism and is soothing and relaxing on the mind. Green appeals to dieters. It helps to alleviate depression and anxiety and is a good choice for anti-aging. Blue and the blue/violet shades produce a calming effect, lowering blood pressure, heart rate and respiration. Blue has a cooling effect in a hot environment.

All the food is organic and freshly prepared by a happy and loving chef. This happiness and blessings are transferred to your being through the food served to you. The server also blesses the food as it is presented to your table.

Eating is never hurried. Each bite of the food is simply an experience of enlightenment. As you feed the body and the mind, you also are feeding the soul. The whole experience is very Zen. When eating you simply experience the joy of eating.

After the meal there is a time to relax, meditate and give thanks. The bill arrives and of course you pay. It is rewarding to pay for the service of another. As you begin to leave you realize that you are now in a state of serenity and peace. You have found enlightenment through practicing Anna-maya-kosha-yoga, the yoga of eating for health and balance, and you have now found a little respite for the hectic and hurried world.

IN CLOSING

As a nutritionist, Naturopathic Doctor and yoga therapist I have worked with numerous clients, been published and lectured to numerous audiences on the effects of diet and practiced yoga for over 30 years. I continually maintain that food and the place it has regarding our health and active lifestyles is the surest way to achieve a life of balanced health and serenity.

When food is prepared lovingly, with only the freshest of ingredients and a focus on vitamins, minerals and nutrition, even the fussiest of us will find eating a pleasurable and rewarding experience.

There is a moment of truth in each human's life. It is a moment when enlightenment has the potential to be realized. For those who grasp the intensity of the moment, they realize it is the beginning of a journey that leads to health, peace and joy.

You are a result of what you think, speak and do. It is so easy for us to get distracted and pay no heed to the blessings and bounties of our lives. We get so caught up in the race to win, to achieve and to attain, often at a cost to our health and our peace of mind.

It is not simply enough to become aware. You must become aware and then move forward with the awareness through the choices and decisions of life. You begin to realize that as you choose to do no harm and focus on what is good and healthy you are able to live without guilt, fear, deceit, greed, anger and pride. You will find that as you organize and support your internal self so will your external self unfold.

The essence of enlightenment is self-balancing. You learn to elevate yourself through the realization that you can improve. Not because things are bad, but because we can always strive to grow and evolve and this means to move from ignorance to awareness. Choosing to balance and support your internal body-mind through healthy and supportive foods brings both strength and gentleness to you.

Anna-maya-kosha yoga not only teaches the yoga of healthy eating, but also teaches us to guard our thoughts and our actions. What we think, speak and do is what we become. As our thoughts enter our minds it is the wise and healthy soul that chooses which thoughts to hang onto and which thoughts to dismiss. That which you elevate and honor is that which you become.

If you choose to honor and elevate the body and the mind through healthy thoughts than what will manifest is healthy actions. These healthy actions will create a life of wisdom revealing to you the ever abundance of life. On the path to enlightenment, one cannot but live the healthy life. This is because we learn to revere all of life. We learn to honor the self through the path of Anna-maya-kosha yoga, which encourages you to inspect what and how you eat. After all, you are, as it is said in Anna yoga; what and how you eat.

When life is seen as a gift the consciousness freely chooses that which is meaningful over that which is meaningless. Joy and happiness founded in a healthy attitude bring balance into your being. This balance is the basis for clarity and truth.

What is the enlightenment found in Anna-maya-kosha- yoga? It is the lightness found within your heart, in the present moment, as you discover that honoring yourself through a healthy lifestyle will open your awareness, so that you are now a little calmer, a bit more balanced, a little bit happier and a little wiser than you were a moment ago.

**You are what and how you eat,
so honor the most important thing in your life;
your health body, mind and soul.**

*Om shanti, shanti, shanti – may this sacred blessing
bring serenity and health to the body,
quietude and peace to the mind, and balanced joy to the soul.*

~ Namaste ~

May you always go with health, happiness and peace

Doctor Lynn

MEAL PLAN

The following meal plans and recipes are only samples. They are not meant to be followed rigidly, but rather to give you a guideline for developing a healthy and balanced meal plan. Use the recipes in the next section of the book to prepare and enjoy dishes that are healthy, balanced, and prepared with joy and peace. Many of these recipes I developed and perfected over the years. I have included some of my children's favorites.

"Let food be thy medicine."
~ Hippocrates circa 431 B.C.~

DAY 1

Breakfast
- ½ cup Granola with 1 ½ tablespoons kefir and sliced banana
- Green tea with or without honey or stevia
- 1 - 4 oz glass of fresh squeezed orange juice

Mid morning
- Small apple

Lunch
- Tuna salad on a bed of organic mixed greens and sliced tomatoes
- Pineapple slices
- Water, herbal tea or green tea

Dinner
- Tandori Salmon
- Steamed broccoli
- Rice pudding
- Water or herbal tea

Evening snack
- Sliced fruit and tea

DAY 2

Breakfast
- Green tea or herbal tea with or without honey, or stevia
- 1 slice of whole grain toast with 1 tablespoon of peanut butter
- 1 - 4 oz glass of fresh squeezed fruit juice

Mid morning snack
- Apple

Lunch
- Natural Yogi salad
- Sliced strawberries
- Herbal tea, water, green tea

Dinner
- Chicken tomasi
- Couscous
- Steamed carrots and broccoli
- Layered fruit salad

DAY 3

Breakfast
- Vegetable and goat cheese omelet
- Sliced kiwi
- Green tea or herbal tea with or without honey or stevia
- 1 - 4 oz glass of fresh squeezed juice

Mid morning
- Banana

Lunch
- Bowl of ready-made organic soup from the health food store
- 1 slice of whole grain bread with ½ tablespoon peanut butter
- Apple
- Water or tea

Dinner
- Marinated tofu
- Basmati rice
- Steamed vegetables – onion, broccoli, yellow squash
- Baked Ricotta with strawberries
- Water or tea

Use the above meal plan as a guide. Each day you should get the right proportion of protein to complex carbohydrates, as well as adequate servings of fruits and vegetables. To eat like a yogi simply remove the processed, refined, denatured, left over foods from your life and learn to eat whole, fresh, and clean foods. Good nutrition is about life enrichment and well-being. In yoga it is taught; that which you honor and elevate is what you become.

In Anna-maya-kosha-yoga it is taught; that which you eat and how you eat is what you become. Honor yourself first by giving yourself the gift of healthy nutrition. It will bring to the body, the mind and the soul the vital energy of life. What could be more precious than a healthy life?

I hope you enjoy the following recipes. Check out my second book in this series; Recipes for Health, Sex, Happiness and Love …eating your way to success.

Recipes

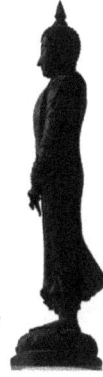

* Some recipes will give approximate calorie intake, protein and carbohydrates in grams

Breakfast

ASPARAGUS AND TOMATO OMELET

Makes 2 servings

- 3 eggs beaten
- ¼ cup non-fat cottage cheese
- 1/3-cup raw blanched asparagus tips
- 1 medium tomato sliced

In a blender or food processor, at medium to high speed, whip eggs and cottage cheese. Heat a skillet with a drizzle of olive oil and pour in the egg mixture. Stir until set. Turn onto a serving plate and arrange asparagus tips and sliced tomatoes on top of the eggs.

LEMON OMELET WITH PAPAYA

Makes 1 serving

- 2 eggs
- 1 teaspoon of honey
- ½ teaspoon grated lemon rind
- ¼ teaspoon vanilla extract
- ¼ papaya seeded and sliced
- Watercress sprigs for garnish

Beat the eggs with the honey, lemon rind, and vanilla until well combined. Pour the mixture in an omelet pan or medium size skillet coated with a natural no-stick spray.

Cook over medium heat, pulling the edges of the omelet towards the center of the pan with a table knife and swirling the pan to allow uncooked eggs to reach the edge.

When the eggs are cooked and just set on top, remove form heat. Lay two slices of papaya down the center of the omelet, fold the omelet over the papaya and slide the omelet out of the pan on to a plate. Garnish with the remaining papaya slices and watercress, if desired.

Calories 261   protein 15 g   carbohydrates 16g

PEANUT BUTTER FRENCH TOAST

Makes 1 serving

- 1 egg
- 1 tablespoon of water
- ¼ of a packet of stevia * herbal sweetener that is sold as a supplement in health food stores
- 2 slices of whole grain bread
- 1 tablespoon of peanut butter
- 1 tablespoon of raisins

In a shallow bowl, combine eggs, water, stevia and beat with a fork. Make a sandwich with the bread, peanut butter and raisins. Dip the sandwich in the egg mixture; turn carefully until the egg is absorbed. Cook sandwich on a preheated nonstick griddle or skillet, over medium heat, turning occasionally, until brown on both sides.

Calories 294   protein 13g   carbohydrates 25g

CINNAMON YOGURT MUFFINS

Makes 8 servings

- 1/-½ cups of whole-wheat flour – or any other whole grain flour
- 1/ ½ teaspoons double acting baking powder
- ¾ teaspoon baking soda
- 2 teaspoons ground cinnamon
- ¼ teaspoon ground nutmeg
- 1/8-teaspoon sea salt
- 1 egg
- ½ cup plain non-fat yogurt
- 2 tablespoons of safflower oil or olive oil
- 1 ½ teaspoon vanilla extract
- 5 packets of stevia

Preheat the oven to 400. In a medium bowl, combine flour, baking powder, baking soda, cinnamon, nutmeg, and salt.

In a larger bowl, combine the remaining ingredients. Beat on low speed of an electric beater until moistened. Divide batter evenly into 8 nonstick muffin cups, or ones that have been sprayed with a nonstick cooking spray.

Bake for 12 minutes until lightly browned. Remove muffins to a rack to cool or serve hot.

Calories 146   protein 4g   carbohydrates 5g

THREE GRAIN PEANUT BUTTER BREAD

Taste great sliced, toasted and served with honey.

- 8 servings
- Preheat over to 350 degrees
- ½ cup of cornmeal
- ½ cup of oatmeal
- 1 cup of whole wheat or any other whole grain flour
- 3 teaspoons of baking powder
- ½ teaspoon of cinnamon
- 1/3 cup of peanut butter
- 2 egg whites
- 1 teaspoon of safflower oil or olive oil
- 1 tablespoon of non-fat yogurt
- 2 packets of stevia
- 1 cup of cold water

In a bowl combine cornmeal, oatmeal, flour, baking powder and cinnamon. Add stevia, peanut butter, egg whites, yogurt and oil. Mix with a fork until blended. Add water and mix thoroughly. Place in nonstick loaf pan and cook for 30 minutes. Allow to cool, removing from pan and serve.

Calories 149   protein 6g   carbohydrates 8g

FRUIT AND KEFIR

- Slice 1 banana in a soup bowl. Add 1 cup sliced melon.
- Top with 2 tablespoons of kefir.
- Top with 1 scoop of soy/whey protein powder.
- Sprinkle ¼ teaspoon of cinnamon on top.
- Melon can be replaced with a pear, apple or any other fruit or berry.

PROTEIN SHAKE

- 1 frozen banana
- 2 tablespoons of kefir
- 1 tablespoon of water
- ¼ cup of berries – strawberries, blackberries, blueberries or combination
- ½ teaspoon cinnamon

Combine in blender and blend into a smoothie.

GRANOLA

Buy all-natural granola from the health food store – without any sugar or preservatives.

- 1 serving of granola
- Add ¼ cup of diced fruit – banana, strawberries, and blueberries
- Pour over top -2 tablespoons of kefir
- 1- 4 oz glass of fresh squeezed juice
- Green tea plain or with honey or stevia

* Exchange granola for oatmeal or any other whole grain cereal that is free of sugar and preservatives.

Appetizers

We often think of Yogis as being reclusive. However, socializing and sharing is a big part of the experience and growth along the spiritual path. As you reach out to share with others try offering these easy and healthy appetizers.

ARTICHOKE SPREAD

- 1 oz can of artichoke hearts
- 1 teaspoon of minced garlic
- 2 teaspoons of chopped scallion
- 1 tablespoon of Dijon mustard
- 1/3 cup low fat shredded parmesan cheese
- Paprika to sprinkle on top

Place all ingredients accept the cheese into a food processor or blender and process until grainy consistency. Hand mix in the cheese. Place in an over proof ceramic or glass dish; sprinkle paprika on top and bake uncovered in 350-degree oven for 15-20 minutes. Serve hot to spread on raw vegetables or slices of pita bread.

Artichokes are an alkaline food and a great source of fiber. Contains vitamin A and C, calcium and iron. Artichokes an excellent elimination food, helping the bowls to move effectively and are therefore good on a reducing diet.

GUACAMOLE DIP

This dip is made with asparagus to reduce the calories and fat of the avocado. However, you can use an avocado in place of the asparagus.

- 1 bunch of steamed asparagus spears – steamed to soft (or 1 large avocado)
- 2 scallions chopped (including some of the green)
- 1 teaspoon of minced garlic
- ¼ cup of jalapeno salsa
- 2 heaping tablespoons of low-fat cottage cheese

Place all ingredients in a blender and blend until smooth. Chill in refrigerator. Serve as a cold dip with raw vegetables.

Replacing the avocado with the asparagus gives this dip a unique taste, saves calories and fat. Asparagus is an alkaline food, stimulating the kidneys, contains chlorophyll so is a good blood builder and is high in vitamin A. Asparagus is a good source of water content and is considered a good vegetable for an eliminating diet.

Avocado is a high and valuable fruit oil. It contains fourteen minerals, which help to regulate body functions and stimulate growth. It also contains sodium and potassium, which give it a PH balancing effect.

HUMMUS SPREAD

This Middle Eastern spread is high in vegetable protein. Beans such as chickpeas are low in fat and high in potassium, iron, thiamine and sodium. Beans are also a great source of complex carbohydrates. The digestive process of beans appears to release protease inhibitors which scientist believe are extremely effective in blocking the formation of certain cancer cells including colon and breast cancer.

- 6 oz can rinse and drained chickpeas (garbanzo beans)
- 2 tablespoons of lemon juice
- 1 tablespoon of tahini (sesame paste)
- 1 teaspoon of olive oil
- 1 teaspoon of minced garlic
- 2 tablespoons of finely minced scallion (green and white portion)
- Dash of paprika

In food processor combine all ingredients accept scallions and paprika and process until pureed. Stir in scallions. Place in serving bowl and chill for 1 hour. Sprinkle top with paprika.

Serve as a salad atop greens and chopped vegetables or serve with slices of pita bread.

Serves 4

PESTO

Pesto is a great garnish for fish, chicken or pasta. It also works well as a dip for raw vegetables

- 1-cup low fat cottage cheese
- 1-cup fresh basil leaves
- 2 tablespoons grated Parmesan cheese
- 1-tablespoon pine nuts or walnuts
- 2 garlic cloves peeled (or use the equivalent minced garlic

In a food processor combine all ingredients and process until smooth. Serve at room temperature or chill.

PESTO DRESSING

- ¾ cup reduced calorie/nondairy mayonnaise (can be found in health food store)
- ½ cup fresh basil leaves
- 2 tablespoon red wine vinegar
- 1 garlic clove peeled (or equivalent minced garlic
- 1-tablespoon pine nuts (or walnuts) chopped

Blend all ingredients accept for nuts in a blender.
Add nuts and use as a dressing.

Makes a great dressing to use on a salad of mixed greens, on top of cooked chicken or fish.

Salads

Just about every culture has some form of salad. Nothing could be better for you than a good mix of greens and vegetables toped with a healthy dressing. This is probably the best way to insure you get your daily allotment of fresh vegetables.

A salad can be an appetizer, a side dish, a snack or a main meal. Here are some unusual healthy salads and dressings. Get creative with fresh fruits and vegetables and take the ordinary to the extraordinary.

The main stay of most salads is the lettuce or greens. The American dinner salad is often made with iceberg lettuce, which is a nutritional washout. Try the following in your salad for nutritional energy and great taste. Dandelion green is high is fiber, calcium, vitamin A and iron. Spinach has more potassium, magnesium and folate in a 2-cup serving than 25% of the recommended RDA. Watercress provides a punch of vitamin C. Arugula is rich in calcium and magnesium making it an excellent bone builder. Bibb lettuce provides energy and folate. Red leaf lettuce has little vitamins C, A and folate so use it to toss in with other greens. Escarole is high in vitamin A. Radicchio is a red leaf lettuce that adds potassium and a splash of color. Belgian endives are high in fiber and work well as a party dippers for healthy appetizers.

One of my favorites is lamb's lettuce also known as mache (rhymes with posh) A three ounces serving provides 100 percent of your daily vitamin A and half of your vitamin C. It's also high in folate and lutien, which are cancer fighting nutrients.

WALDORF SALAD

- 1 cup of plain organic nonfat yogurt
- ¼ cup of reduced fat non-dairy mayonnaise
- 2 teaspoons of lemon juice
- 1 packet of stevia
- 4 small sweet apples diced and peeled
- 1 cup chopped celery
- 1 tablespoon of sunflower seeds
- ½ cup chopped walnuts
- Shredded bib lettuce

Place yogurt, mayonnaise, lemon juice and stevia in a bowl and mix. Add remaining ingredients (accept bibb lettuce) and toss. Chill to blend flavors. Serve over bibb lettuce. In many ancient cultures the walnut was thought to bring good luck and good health. The Romans called the walnut the 'royal' nut. The oil found in walnuts is one of the 'good guys', polyunsaturated fats which tends to lower cholesterol.

Serves 4

Calories 158   Protein 5g   Carbohydrates 23g

SPINACH SALAD

Fresh spinach greens are delicious way to get your daily dosage of potassium, magnesium and folate.

- ½ package of fresh spinach – remove stems and rinse
- 1 small 8-ounce package of fresh mushrooms – sliced and rinsed
- 2 shallots sliced into rings

Arrange mushrooms and shallots atop a bed of spinach
Drizzle over the top:
Combine in a jar and shake well –
- 1 tablespoon of olive oil
- 1 tablespoon plus one teaspoon of wine vinegar
- 1/8 teaspoon of garlic salt
- 2 teaspoons of Dijon mustard

Serves two

SPINACH-STRAWBERRY SALAD

Wash fresh spinach and remove the stems.

- 1/3 cup of reduced fat non-dairy mayonnaise
- ¼ cup fresh squeezed orange juice
- ½ packet of stevia
- 1 teaspoon of poppy seeds (or sesame seeds)
- ½ pound fresh spinach
- 2 cups of sliced fresh strawberries

Combine first four ingredients in a bowl; stir well and set aside. Gently toss spinach and strawberries in a large bowl and arrange on 8 salad plates. Drizzle 1 tablespoon of the dressing over each salad. Strawberries are an excellent source of fiber and vitamin C. They make an excellent spring tonic as an alkaline food they help the body to maintain balance. Serves 8 – about 54 calories per serving.

APPLE, PEAR, AND BLUEBERRY SALAD

*3 tablespoons of fresh mint vinegar –
Place 1 cup of fresh chopped mint leaves in a large bowl. Pour 2 cups of white wine vinegar into a medium saucepan; bring to a boil, and pour over the mint. Let stand for 30 minutes. Strain mixture; discard mint. Yields two cups at about 3 calories per tablespoon.

SALAD

- 3 tablespoons of fresh mint vinegar
- 2 tablespoons of water
- 1 tablespoon of olive oil
- ½ teaspoon of Dijon mustard
- ½ teaspoon of honey
- 1/8 teaspoon of sea salt
- 2 cups of shredded Boston lettuce
- 1 cup torn watercress
- 4 Boston lettuce leaves
- 1 medium sized red delicious apple cored and thinly sliced
- 1 medium pear cored and thinly sliced
- ½ cup fresh blueberries
- 2 teaspoons of chopped fresh mint

Combine first 6 ingredients in a small bowl, stirring with a wire whisk until blended. Combine shredded lettuce and watercress in a medium bowl. Pour ¼ cup vinegar mixture over greens, tossing gently. Arrange lettuce on a serving platter; spoon tossed greens on lettuce leaves. Arrange apple and pear slices alternately on leaves. Sprinkle blueberries and mint evenly over salad. Drizzle remaining vinegar mixture over fruit. Yields 4 servings.

About 93 calories per serving,   Protein .8g   carbohydrates 15.2g

MACHE SALAD — LAMB'S LETTUCE

- 4 ounces of mache lettuce
- 2 avocados skinned, pitted and cut into chunks
- 2 grapefruit. Peeled and sectioned, drain and reserve the juice
- ½ cup roasted, chopped macadamia nuts (use almonds or walnuts)

CITRUS VINAIGRETTE

- 1-tablespoon grapefruit juice
- 1-tablespoon lime juice
- Grated zest of one lime
- 2 tablespoons extra virgin olive oil
- Dash of sea salt and a dash of black pepper

Whisk vinaigrette ingredients together. Toss with mache, avocado, grapefruit sections and toasted macadamia nuts.

Serves 4

Mache can be combined with other greens to make a salad. It's a sweet leafy green that is high in folate lutein and vitamin C.

SPINACH AND ARUGULA SALAD

- ½ pound spinach – washed stems removed
- ¼ pound of arugula
- 6 medium mushrooms thinly sliced

Toss together in a bowl.

Stir together:
- 1 tablespoons Dijon mustard
- 4 teaspoons of dark sesame oil
- 1 tablespoon of apple cider vinegar
- 1 teaspoon of honey
- 1 tablespoon of chopped chives
- Dash of sea salt and a dash of black pepper

Toast 1 tablespoon of sesame seeds in a small skillet over medium heat until lightly brown. Toss the greens with the dressing and then sprinkle the sesame seeds on top.

Serves 4

MARINATED ARTICHOKE HEARTS

- 1 cup canned artichoke hearts, drained
- 1/8 teaspoon of garlic powder
- 1 tablespoon plus 1 teaspoon of olive oil
- 2 tablespoons of red wine vinegar
- ¼ teaspoon of sea salt
- ¼ teaspoon of oregano
- ¼ teaspoon of dry mustard
- ½ packet of stevia
- Dash of black pepper

Combine all ingredients in a bowl. Cover and refrigerate for several hours or overnight, stirring occasionally.

Serve cold – serves 4
Calories 58   Protein 1g   carbohydrates 5g

COTTAGE CHEESE DIP

- 1-cup low fat cottage cheeses
- 1-tablespoon low-fat non-dairy mayonnaise
- 2 tablespoons of chopped dill pickles
- 1 tablespoon of chopped pimento
- 1 tablespoon of chopped chives

In mixing bowl mix together cottage cheese and mayonnaise. Stir in other ingredients and chill.
Serve with raw vegetables or slices of endives for dippers.
Makes about 1/1/4 cups of dip at about 16 calories per tablespoon.

*Quick Salad side dish

CARROT AND ALFALFA SPROUT SALAD

Use a food processor to shred three large carrots. Toss with 1 cup of alp alfalfa sprouts. Sprinkle with a dash of sea salt and a dash of black pepper. Squeeze the juice of one lemon over the top and serve.

Serves 6   Approximately 20 calories per serving

TANGY CUCUMBER SALAD

- 1 tablespoon Dijon mustard
- ¼ cup of plain kefir
- 1 cup of cucumber very thinly sliced

Stir mustard and kefir in a bowl. Gently stir in cucumbers.
Refrigerate for several hours
Serves 2   35 calories per serving

CRANBERRY – ORANGE RELISH

- 1 12-ounce bag of fresh cranberries
- 4 oranges – cut off ends, slice with the peel into 4 or 5 slices
- 2 packets of stevia

Place in a food processor and chop well. Chill for 24 hours. Use as a garnish – place on top of parsley for decoration. Great with meat or poultry.

CRANBERRY VINAIGRETTE

- 1 12-ounce bag of cranberries
- 4 cups of rice wine vinegar and
- 2 packets of stevia

Simmer cranberries with vinegar and stevia for 5 minutes until the cranberries pop. Let stand to cool. Pour through a fine strainer into a clean quart bottle. Use over salads.

PINEAPPLE SLAW

- 2 cups of shredded cabbage
- ¼ cup diced green pepper
- ½ cup canned crushed pineapple (unsweetened) drained
- 2 tablespoons of apple cider vinegar
- ¼ cup low-fat non-dairy mayonnaise
- 2 teaspoons of minced onions
- ¼ teaspoon of curry powder
- ¼ teaspoon of celery seed

Combine cabbage, green pepper and pineapple in a large bowl. Toss to combine. Stir vinegar into mayonnaise in a small bowl. Stir in seasonings. Pour over cabbage mixture. Toss to blend well. Chill and toss before serving.

Serves 4   about 75 calories
Protein 1g   carbohydrates 4g

Always use fresh ingredients in salads. Mix the greens and vegetables along with the following dressing suggestions

Ever since Biblical times, Cilantro has been called the 'healer from heaven'. It's recommended for indigestion, flatulence, and diarrhea. Scientists have discovered that it has anti-inflammatory properties and that it can help to reduce blood sugar levels. Here is an easy relish that can be used as a salad dressing or served with grilled chicken or fish to add flavor.

CILANTRO RELISH

- 1 cup chopped cilantro leaves
- 1 clove garlic
- ½ tsp cumin
- ½ tsp sea salt
- 1 Tablespoon cider vinegar
- 8 ounces non-fat plain yogurt or kefir

Mash together garlic, cumin, salt and vinegar. Add cilantro and yogurt and stir. *Option- add some chopped walnuts

Use balsamic vinegar to sprinkle over the top of salads and vegetables. Mix it with 2 parts olive oil for a fragrant salad dressing. Mix with Dijon mustard as a great sauce for cooking chicken and fish. Sprinkle over strawberries, raspberries, peaches or melon for an unusual fresh fruit dessert.

Combine apple cider vinegar with a little honey and oil for a sweet and sour dressing and sauce.

Use mustard mixed with a little honey as a dressing or sauce for cooking.

HERBED KEFIR DRESSING

- 1 tablespoon plus 1 teaspoon olive oil
- 1-cup plain kefir
- 2 tablespoons red wine vinegar
- ½ teaspoon oregano
- ½ teaspoon of dill weed
- 1/8 teaspoon of garlic powder
- 1 tablespoon minced onion
- Dash of seas salt and a dash of black pepper

Stir oil into kefir. Add remaining ingredients. Mix well. Chill to blend flavors. Stir before serving. Use as a dressing for salads or as a marinate for chicken or vegetables.

Lunch Salads

BASIC TOFU SALAD

* also see tofu recipes for additional salads and spreads

- 1 pound of hard tofu
- 1 tablespoon of olive oil
- 1-teaspoon fresh lemon juice
- 1 teaspoon grated garlic
- ½ teaspoon of onion powder
- ¼ cup finely chopped parsley
- 1 teaspoon of mustard
- Dash of seas salt and dash of black pepper

Chop the tofu finely and combine with the remaining ingredients. Let sit for 30 minutes and taste. Makes three cups of salad. Serve on a sandwich or on a bed of greens.

Optional additions:
- ¼ chopped dilled pickle
- ¼ cup diced celery
- ¼ cup diced tomato
- 1 Tablespoon minced green onion
- 2 teaspoons chopped capers
- 1 tablespoon chopped olives
- ¼ cup chopped cilantro

BLACK BEAN AND PEPPER SALAD

- 1 16-ounce can of black beans
- 1 green bell pepper
- ½ jalapeno pepper
- 1 lime
- 2 tablespoon chopped red onion
- 2 tablespoons of chopped fresh parsley
- Dash of sea salt and dash of pepper

Drain and rinse the black beans. Chop the green pepper and the jalapeno pepper. Grate the green zest form the lime and squeeze 1 tablespoon 1 of juice. Combine all the ingredients and toss lightly

Serves 4   90 calories per serving

Protein 6g   carbohydrates 15g

TUNA SALAD

Start with a six-ounce can of water packed tuna drained and add the following for variations:

To tuna add 2 tablespoons of low-fat non-dairy mayonnaise, 1 tablespoon each of chopped rosemary and chopped capers. Dash with freshly ground black pepper. Mound tuna on bread add lettuce and sliced tomato

Instead of mayonnaise add ¼ cup of ricotta cheeses. Season with salt and pepper. Spread on bread or pile on lettuce greens and top with roasted red pepper and fresh basil leaves.

Make tuna salad with mayonnaise or ricotta. Spread the bread with a thin layer of olive paste (mash black or green olives into a paste). Top with tomato slices and fresh basil.

Add Dijon or honey mustard to tuna and mayonnaise to give tuna a sweet and sour effect. Add a splash of balsamic vinegar.

WARM WALNUT SALAD
WITH CRANBERRY AND ORANGE DRESSING

- 4 ounces of organic mixed greens
- 1 leek sliced ¼ inch crosswise and then washed
- ¼ cup chopped walnuts
- 1 tablespoon of olive oil
- 2 teaspoons of cranberry vinaigrette * see dressing recipes above
- Zest of one orange grated finely
- 2 ounces of goat cheese crumbled and cut into pieces
- Sea salt and black pepper to taste

Pour olive oil in a sauté pan over medium heat and sauté leek until brown. Add walnuts and continue to sauté for 2 minutes. Remove pan form burner. Add Vinaigrette and orange zest to the warm pan and let sit for 20 seconds. Top lettuce with goat cheese salt and pepper. Pour contents of pan over the goat cheeses and lettuce. Toss to serve.

The secret to this dish is that it is served warm. Try using Roquefort cheese in place of goat cheese. Garnish the top with more orange zest. As a main meal add grilled chicken or grilled salmon and orange slices.
Serves 2

ROASTED BEET, ONION AND GOAT CHEESE SALAD

- 3 cups of balsamic vinegar
- 2 pounds trimmed baby beets – a mixture of red and golden
- olive oil
- Black peeper
- 1 ½ pounds large red or yellow sweet onions (or combination of the two)
- ¾ cups of large black olives
- 8 ounces of organic mixed greens
- 6 ounces of goat cheese sliced

Gently boil the 3 cups of balsamic vinegar for 20 – 30 minutes or until it is reduced to about ½ cup. Store at room temperature.

Wash beets well to remove the dirt. Preheat oven to 375 degrees. Place beets on roasting pan and toss with olive oil to coat lightly. Season with seas salt and black pepper and roast for 30-40 minutes or until tender. Remove from oven and let the beets cool. Rub off skins with paper towel and slice. Set aside.

While beets are roasting peel and cut the red or yellow onion into thick wedges. Lightly brush with olive oil and season with sea salt and black pepper. Place in a single layer-roasting pan along with the olives and roast at 375 for 20 minutes. Set aside.

To serve arrange greens on a plate and top with beets, onions, olives and a slice of goat cheese. Drizzle a few drops of olive oil and reduced balsamic vinegar over the top of the salad.

Serves 6   278 calories   protein 10g   carbohydrates 24g

HERBED CHICKEN SALAD

Sprinkle boneless chicken breast or thigh (8oz per serving) with sea salt and black pepper. Broil and slice.

Combine 2 tablespoons of low-fat non-dairy mayonnaise and 2 tablespoons of fresh lemon juice with 1 tablespoon each of chopped fresh basil ands chopped fresh mint. Serve over a bed of organic mixed greens.

Serves one – double recipe for each additional 8 ounce serving of chicken

MANGO LIME SALSA CHICKEN SALAD

Rub boneless chicken thigh or breast (8 ounce) with ½ teaspoon of chili powder and broil. Slice. Combine 1 cup diced fresh mango and 2 teaspoons each of honey, lime juice and minced scallions. Place sliced chicken over a bed of organic mixed greens and pour salsa over the top.

CRANBERRY CHICKEN

Rub 8-ounce boneless chicken thigh or breast with 1 teaspoon of crumbled rosemary. Broil. Combine ½ cup of cranberry relish * see recipe above- with 1 teaspoon of minced crystallized ginger. Serve over a bed of organic mixed greens. Garnish with orange slices.

WARM GREEK CHICKEN SALAD

- 1 pound of boneless chicken breast cut into bite size pieces
- ¼ teaspoon of seas salt
- 2 cups of broccoli flowerets
- 2 cups of cauliflower flowerets
- 1 medium size carrot cut diagonally into ¼ inch thick slices
- 2 eggs beaten
- 2 tablespoon of lemon juice
- 1/8 teaspoon of black pepper
- Chopped parsley

Place chicken and vegetables in a steamer basket or colander and place in a sauce pan of simmering water. Cover and simmer for 7 minutes and simmer over medium heat until tender. Remove chicken and vegetables to platter and keep warm.

Strain ½ cup broth from saucepan. Beat together the eggs and lemon juice in a small saucepan. Stir in the ½ cup of broth and pepper. Cook over low heat, stirring until sauce thickens (about 2 minutes)- do not boil. Spoon the warm sauce over the vegetables and chicken and garnish with parsley.

229 calories per serving   serves 4

protein 33g   Carbohydrates   14g

Soups

Nothing warms the body, mind and soul like a hot bowl of nourishing soup. Soup is also a great way to watch your weight as it is filling and satisfying without a lot of heavy and rich calories.

VEGETABLE SOUP

- 3-½ cups water
- 1-tablespoon chicken flavored bouillon granules
- 1 (14 ½ -ounce) can- no salt whole tomatoes, un-drained and chopped
- ¼ cup minced onion
- 1 teaspoon of dried whole basil
- 1 teaspoon of paprika
- ¾ teaspoon instant minced garlic
- ¼ teaspoon of seas salt
- 1 cup sliced carrots
- 1 cup of sliced fresh mushrooms
- 1 cup diced zucchini
- 2 tablespoons of burgundy or other red wine

Combine water, bouillon, tomatoes, onion, basil, paprika, garlic, and salt in Dutch oven. Bring to a boil; cover, reduce heat and simmer for 10 minutes. Add carrots; cover and simmer for 10 minutes. Add mushrooms, zucchini and wine and simmer uncovered for 8 minutes.

* Options add 1 cup of diced cooked chicken with mushrooms and zucchini for chicken vegetable soup.
*

Serve 7   protein 6.8g   carbohydrates 9.5 g

PUMPKIN CURRY SOUP

- 1 small onion finely chopped
- 1 small green pepper finely chopped
- ½ of a 16-ounce can of unseasoned pumpkin puree
- 1 – 14.5 ounce can of chicken broth or use vegetable broth
- 1 teaspoon of curry powder
- 2 tablespoons of fresh chopped parsley
- 1 teaspoon of olive oil
- Non-fat plain yogurt
- Crushed red pepper

In medium saucepan over medium heat sauté onion and pepper in olive oil for about 2 minutes. Add pumpkin puree and chicken broth. Stir with wire Wisk until smooth. Heat to boiling, stirring constantly. Stir in the curry and parsley. Pour into individual bowls. Place a tablespoon of yogurt in the center of each and swirl. Sprinkle the top with crushed red pepper.

Serves 2   120 calories each

SEAFOOD CREOLE

- ¼ cup chopped onion
- ¼ cup chopped green pepper
- 1 cup low fat cottage cheese
- 1 –16 ounce can stew tomatoes
- 1 cup of water
- 1 package of chicken flavored bouillon
- 1 teaspoon of oregano
- dash of cayenne pepper

- ½ teaspoon of minced garlic
- ½ pound of cooked flaky white fish such as Pollock or haddock
- ½ pound of fresh cooked and cleaned shrimp or ½ pound of lobster meat chopped into small bite size pieces

Pour 2 tablespoons of water in a pan, add onion, green pepper and minced garlic, sauté.

In a blender or food processor bled other ingredients except for the fish and shrimp. Add to the sautéed vegetables. Heat to simmer but do not boil. Add fish and seafood and continue to simmer. Divided into 4 even bowls. Sprinkle the top with fresh chopped parsley.
Note: may be served over a bed of rice
Serves 4 125 calories each

MISO SOUP

Miso is a paste made form fermented soybeans. It provides enzymes and cleanses toxins from the body. Be careful not to boil the Miso as that will destroy the enzymes Miso comes in a variety of flavors. Dark reds are best for fall and winter while the lighter colors are best for spring and summer.

- 1 (5-inch piece kombu sea vegetable
- 6 cups of water
- 2 dried shiitake mushrooms
- 3 tablespoons of white or red miso
- 2 green onions chopped
- slivered lemon rind
- ¼ cup diced tofu

Bring the kombu and mushrooms to a boil in the water, then lower the heat and simmer for 15 minutes. Strain the broth. Bring the dashi (broth) to a boil, and then turn off the heat and add tofu. In a cup dissolve the Miso in 3 tablespoons of the hot stock and add to the dashi.

Ladle the Miso soup into 6 bowls and garnish each with chopped green onion and slivered lemon rid. Variation- garnish with thinly sliced mushrooms and seaweed.

Serves 6   37 calories each
Protein 2g   carbohydrates   7g

CHICKEN CALYPSO SOUP

- 2 tablespoons of olive oil
- 1 cup chopped onion
- 1 clove of garlic minced
- ½ teaspoon of curry powder
- ¾ pound boneless skinless chicken breast or thighs cut into ½ inch pieces
- 1 teaspoon of Dijon mustard
- 2 - 14-ounce cans of low sodium chicken broth
- 1 - 8-ounce can of unsweetened crushed pineapple in juice un-drained
- ground black pepper
- ½ cup chopped fresh spinach
- 3 kiwi fruits
- ½ cup shredded toasted coconut

In large skillet over medium heat sauté onion, garlic and curry powder in oil. Stir in chicken and mustard, and cook until slightly brown. Stir in remaining ingredients accept kiwi fruit and coconut. Bring to a boil. Meanwhile peel and slice kiwi into ½ sliced – cut in half. Boil soup for 5 minutes, add kiwi and simmer for 2 more minutes. Ladle soup into 6 bowls and garnish the top with toasted cocoanut.

Serves 6   205 calories each

Vegetable Dishes

RATATOUILLE

Ratatouille is also a soup as well as a vegetable dish. You can also add diced cooked chicken to make it a meat meal. Each of the vegetables in Ratatouille have healing properties; zucchini is good for elimination and healthy skin; red pepper contains copious amounts of vitamin C, the anti-stress vitamin; and eggplant is considered to be the most powerful food for a woman as it is both energizing and soothing.

- 4 large scallions diced (about ½ cup)
- 2 cloves of garlic minced
- 1 medium eggplant peeled
- 1 cup fresh sliced mushrooms
- ½ cup celery chopped
- 2 large tomatoes chopped
- 2 small zucchinis sliced
- 1 sweet red pepper diced
- 2 tablespoons olive oil
- 1 teaspoon of basil
- 1 teaspoon of oregano
- 1 tablespoon of dry white wine
- Dash of dried red pepper

Sauté onion and garlic in olive oil over medium heat. Stir in eggplant, mushrooms and celery and cook for five minutes, stirring occasionally. Stir in tomatoes, zucchini, scallions, oregano, basil, wine and red pepper. Reduce heat to low and simmer for 15 minutes until eggplant is tender. Add a dash of dried red pepper.

Options – add 1 cup of diced cooked chicken or add 1 cup of canned red kidney beans. Serve over basmati rice.

Serve in bowls topped with a little grated Parmesan cheese.
Serves 4   116 calories per serving
Protein 7g   carbohydrates 23g

COACH HOUSE SPINACH

Spinach is one of the top four foods on the ORAC scale, which measures the amount of anti-oxidants in foods.

- 1 pound of fresh spinach – washed with stems removed
- 1 tablespoon of thyme
- ¼ cup of chopped scallions
- ¼ cup shredded carrots
- 1 clove of garlic

Place spinach in a steaming basket over boiling water. Add thyme, scallions and carrots. Push the garlic through a garlic press over the spinach. Cover and steam until the spinach is wilted and bright green.

Serves 4

SUMMER SQUASH WITH GREMOLATA

Steam summer squash to slightly crisp. Dump steaming vegetables into a serving plate and top with gremolata

GREMOLATA

This can be used to top any steamed vegetables or salad.
- 2 tablespoons of minced fresh parsley
- 2 teaspoons grated lemon rind
- 1 small garlic clove minced
- 1/8 teaspoon of black pepper
- Mix together in a bowl and sprinkle over warm vegetables.

Serves 4   29 calories

LEMON BROCCOLI

Recently scientist have found a compound – diindolylmethane, found in cruciferous vegetables 9broccoli, cauliflower, cabbage, Brussels sprouts) that stimulates estrogen metabolism and thus helps with a woman's PMS and menopause as well as helping to prevent breast cancer and uterine cancer. Because it helps with metabolism, it also has applications for weight loss and muscle growth.

- 1 pound of fresh broccoli
- 2 tablespoons of olive oil
- ¼ cup chopped green onion
- ¼ cup chopped celery
- 1 tablespoon plus 1 teaspoon of fresh squeezed lemon juice
- ¼ teaspoon grated lemon rind

Steam fresh broccoli about 10m minutes until tender but still crisp. While broccoli is steaming sauté onion and celery in olive oil. Stir in lemon juice. Place broccoli in a serving dish. Pour onion mixture over the top. Sprinkle with lemon rind.

Serves 4   96 calories
Protein 5g   carbohydrates 9g

ROASTED VEGETABLES

You can use any combination of vegetables for this recipe, however the following is an interesting combination.

- 2 large red bell peppers
- 2 large yellow bell peppers
- 4 medium bulbs fennel
- 3 tablespoon of olive oil
- 4 tablespoons of fresh squeezed orange juice
- 1 tablespoon of finely chopped rosemary
- 1 tablespoon finely chopped marjoram
- Freshly ground black pepper

Trim and cut the fennel bulbs in half. Slice the peppers into quarters, removing seeds and stems. Combine olive oil, orange juice and spices. Marinate vegetables for about 30 minutes.

Place vegetables on a baking sheet and drizzle with the marinate. Roast at 375 degrees for about 25 minutes. Serve warm.
Options – sprinkle top with grated Parmesan cheese.
Serves 6   94 calories per serving
Protein 3g   carbohydrates 21g

Legumes

Simple vegetarian foods such as legumes (beans) in Indian scriptures is referred to as sattvic bhoj which means the pure essence of food. A person who eats sattvic bhoj is said to be more calm, mentally agile and clearer thinking than one who eats heavier foods.

BAKED LENTILS WITH TOMATOES

- 2 tablespoons of olive oil
- ½ cup chopped onions
- ½ cup chopped celery
- ½ cup chopped green pepper
- 1- 16-ounce can tomatoes. Chopped and drained
- ½ teaspoon dried oregano
- Dash of garlic powder
- 16 ounces of cooked lentils
- 2 tablespoons of wheat germ or dried breadcrumbs
- 1 tablespoon grated Parmesan cheese

Heat oil in pan add onion and green pepper and cook until tender. Preheat oven to 350 degrees.

In a 1-½ quart baking dish spray with a non-stick cooking spry. Combine onion mixture with tomatoes, oregano, garlic powder, pepper and lentils. Mix well. Sprinkle top with wheat germ and parmesan cheese. Bake uncovered for 30 minutes.

Serves 4   238 calories   protein 12g   carbohydrates   33g

BAKED BEANS

- 4 cups dried pea or great Northern beans
- 1-teaspoon sea salt
- 2 medium onions peeled
- 4 cloves of garlic
- ½ cup molasses
- 1-cup brown sugar
- 2 teaspoons dry mustard
- 1-teaspoon black pepper
- 2 cups pf water

Put the beans in a large saucepan and pour enough cold water to cover them. Bring to a boil, let boil for two minutes, remove from heat and let the beans soak in hot water for an hour. Bring them to a boil again and let boil for 30 minutes until beans ar3 partially done. Drain and discard the water.

Preheat the oven to 250 degrees. Use a traditional 4-quart bean pot with a top to bake the beans. Place onions -each with a clove of garlic stuck in the middle in the bottom of the pot and cover with the beans. In a small mixing bowl combine the molasses, ¼ cup of the brown sugar, mustard and a teaspoon of salt and pepper. Slowly stir with a large spoon, pour in the two cups of water. Pour the mixture over the beans. Cover and bake in the center of the over for 4 12/ to 5 hours. Bake uncovered for ½ hour and serve.

TOFU

Tofu is one of the most versatile protein foods and has been a staple of the Asian diet for about 2000 years. Also called bean curd, tofu is made by curdling the white 'milk' of the soybean. It is high in protein (complete protein providing all the essential amino acids), low in fat, calories and carbohydrates and contains no cholesterol. Recent medical research indicates that soy protein can help prevent cancer, ease menopause symptoms and help in diabetes and digestive disorders.

Soybean products contain certain enzyme prohibitors and can cause gas and excessive discomfort. The amount of soy products you would need to eat to be adversely affected would exceed the normal dietary intake. Further there is some controversy over the processing of tofu. Buying organic and rinsing it well helps to minimize any adverse effects. Rinsing well and cooking before eating tofu helps to eliminate gas. For those who are lactose intolerant or want to substitute meat and dairy for a plant-based protein, tofu is the natural choice. As a rule, use firm tofu for slicing and dicing and soft tofu for blending. Try this miso dressing to add flavor to salads, sandwiches and hot steamed vegetables.

- 1-tablespoon white or yellow miso
- 2 tablespoons of fresh lemon juice
- 1 tablespoon of sesame seeds
- 1 teaspoon of sesame seed oil
- 2 teaspoons of honey

Combine all ingredients and whisk together. Makes 12 servings at about 15 calories per serving. Variation – use orange or lime juice. Add ginger, garlic, cilantro or mint.

BAKED TOFU

Use 1 block (1 pound) of firm tofu. Rinse and lightly squeeze out the excess water. Slice ¼ to ½ inch thick slices. Use a glass-baking dish. Cover the bottom of the pan with canola oil or canola oil spray. Sprinkle lemon juice over the top of the tofu. Top with soy sauce and bake at 350 degrees for 20 to 40 minutes. The longer the cooking time the crispier or chewier the texture will be.

Option - add to the soy sauce, garlic or onion powder or a sugar free barbeque sauce.

MARINATED TOFU

Slice tofu as described above. Cover glass bottom of pan with oil. Marinate for a least 2 hours in a mixture of ¼ cup soy sauce, ¼ cup water and 1 tablespoon of grated peeled ginger. Garlic may be minced and added to the marinate. Flip tofu once while marinating. Bake at 350 degrees for 30 minutes. Serve with stir fried vegetables.

* or marinate in 1 tablespoon chopped fresh ginger, 1 teaspoon sesame oil, 2 tablespoons wheat free tamari, 2 tablespoons honey

TOFU SALAD

Slice 1-½ pounds of firm tofu into ½ inch thick slices. Sprinkle with lemon juice and bake in a lightly oiled glass dish at 375 degree until medium hard, about 20-25 minutes. Grate when cooled. Meanwhile mix in a bowl.

3 celery sticks diced
2/3 cup grated radish, carrots and zucchini combination
½ sweet red pepper finely chopped

2/3 dilled pickles finely chopped

Add the grated tofu and mix well. Add the following dressing and serve with crackers, bread or on lettuce.

DRESSING

- ¼ -1/2 cup nonfat nondairy mayonnaise
- 1 teaspoon of lemon juice
- ½ teaspoon of sea salt
- 1/2teaspoon of pepper

TOFU SPREAD

Both tofu and sesame seed are high in calcium and protein. Tahini is sesame paste and can be found in health food stores.

- 1-pound firm tofu rinsed and squeezed of excess water.
- 1-2 sticks of celery finely diced
- 1 scallion finely chopped
- 1/8-cup fresh parsley
- 1/8 cup or either finely diced sweet red pepper or finely grated carrot

Steam tofu for 5 to 10 minutes in a steamer. Squeeze out any excess water. Crumble and mash the tofu with the above ingredients.

In a separate bowl mix

- 1 tablespoon lemon juice
- 1/3 –1/2 cups of nondairy nonfat mayonnaise
- 1 ½ tablespoon nutritional yeast flakes – found in health food store
- 1 teaspoon of vegetable seasoning

• 2 tablespoons of sesame tahini

Combine tofu mixture with mayonnaise mixture. Serve with crackers, bread or over a bed of lettuce.

ITALIAN TOFU MEATBALLS

• 15 ounces firm tofu
• 3 tablespoons pasta Seasoning Blends – Trader Joe's non-irradiated blend
• 2 Slices of whole wheat bread crumbled or ½ cup Coaches Oats
• May use bread crumbs or wheat germ
• 1 egg

Sauce:
• 1 –8 ounce can tomato sauce
• 1 teaspoon Pasta Blend – Trader Joe's
• 1 tablespoon of freshly grated Parmesan Cheese

Preheat over to 375 degrees. Slice tofu and drain well between two sheets of paper towels, squeeze out excess water. In large bowl, combine tofu, seasoning, bread and egg. Mix well with a fork, mashing to blend ingredients. Shape mixture into balls, squeezing tightly.

Place "meatballs" in a single layer in a shallow baking pan that has been sprayed with a nonstick cooking spray. In a small bowl, combine sauce ingredients. Spoon over "meatballs." Sprinkle with Parmesan cheese. Bake for 20 minutes.

2 servings   320 calories each
Protein 3g   Carbohydrates   29g

CAULIFLOWER TOFU BAKE

Note can use broccoli or any other vegetable

- 1 medium head of fresh cauliflower – steam flowerets
- 6 – ounces of soft tofu drained and mashes
- 2 ounces of grated Parmesan cheese
- ¼ cup reduced calorie Italian dressing

Place cooked cauliflower in a 1-quart baking dish that has been sprayed with a nonstick cooking spray.

Preheat oven to 375 degrees.

In a small bowl, combine tofu, parmesan cheese and dressing. Mix well. Spoon over cauliflower.

Bake for 20 minutes.

Serves 2   220 calories each

Protein 17g   carbohydrates 9g

Serve with a side salad of mixed greens and sliced tomatoes for a complete vegetarian meal.

See dessert section for more tofu recipes

VEGGIE BURGER WITH PAPAYA SALSA

- 1 16-ounce can of chickpeas (garbanzo beans) drained
- ¼ cup minced cilantro
- 1 clove of garlic minced
- 2 egg whites
- 1 teaspoon of sea salt
- ¼ teaspoon cayenne pepper
- 1/3-cup whole-wheat flour
- 2 tablespoon of olive oil

Process all ingredients except for the flour in a food processor or blender until combined. Place the flour on waxed paper. Drop a fourth of the mixture onto the flour, and using wet fingertips, gently shape into a patty. Flip to coat the other side. Make three more patties. Heat the oil in a large non-stick skillet over medium heat and cook patties until golden on both sides. Serve on whole grain rolls with salsa.

SALSA

- 2 plum tomatoes sliced
- 1 papaya peeled, seeded and diced
- 2 tablespoons apple cider vinegar
- 1 tablespoon of honey
- 1 jalapeno pepper, seeded and minced
- 1- tablespoon lemon juice

Combine all ingredients – makes 2 cups about 40 calories per serving

Rice and Pastas

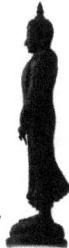

Whole grains - complex carbohydrates - fibers are essential to a healthy and balanced diet. Fiber found in complex carbohydrates not only helps to fill the stomach and make you feel full but also is essential to a healthy digestive track. Whole grains have their bran layer in tact and bran is an important fiber. In addition, whole grains contain the germ or heart of the seed of the grain, which contains important vitamins and minerals. Remember the yoga way is not about losing weight but about eating healthy.

Look for darker grain products and be careful to read labels making sure that whole grains are unprocessed. Choose brown rice over white rice, which has had all the nutrients ground out through a bleaching process. There are many wonderful grains to choose for a healthy diet. I would suggest bulger, barley, jasmine rice, japonica rice, whole wheat pastas, brown rice and basmati rice. Let's look at brown rice and basmati rice, and bulger as great choices.

BASMATI RICE

This naturally whole rice is revered throughout Asia. It is fragrant, high-quality rice that appears in Persia as well as Asian cuisine. Basmati grows white in its natural state, which means it has not been polished or milled and stripped away from most of its vitamin and nutrient content. It is abundant in vitamin B and protein.

- 1-cup basmati rice
- 2 teaspoons of sesame oil
- ½ teaspoon of garam masala
- 1 ½- cups water
- 1 teaspoon of sea salt

Rinse the rice two or three times until the water is clean. Let soak for about 10 minutes and then drain. Heat the oil and garam masala in a skillet and when hot add the rice and stir to coat. Add the water and salt and bring to a boil. Turn the heat down and simmer until most of the water on top of the rice has been absorbed – about 5 minutes. Turn off the heat and let the rice stand, covered for 5 minutes.

Stir in chopped/diced cooked vegetables and/or diced chicken or tofu. Or add raisins and nuts for sweeter rice. Stir-fry or add to any of your favorite dishes.

190 calories 4 servings

Protein 4 g   Carbohydrates 38g

BROWN RICE

Rice is the most consumed food in the world. It is the staple of most diets in many countries. Rice is brown in its natural state. The difference between brown and white rice is found in the outer hull or layer, known as the rice bran, which contains 65 percent of the nutrients found in the rice kernel.

ORIENTAL BROWN FIRED RICE

- 1 tablespoon plus 1 teaspoon of olive oil
- 2 cups of steamed – cooked brown rice
- 2 tablespoons of soy sauce
- Dash of garlic pepper
- Dash of ginger powder
- ½ cup sliced green onions
- 2 eggs - beaten

Heat oil in large skillet over medium heat. Add rice, soy sauce, garlic powder and ginger. Cook, stirring, until rice is hot. Stir in the onions. Cook until onions are tender. Slowly stir in the eggs a little at a time. Cook stirring until eggs are set.

Variation: add 6 ounces of cooked shrimp, diced chicken or tofu before adding the eggs.

Serves 4 269 calories each with shrimp, chicken or tofu
Protein 17g   Carbohydrates 27g

WHOLE WHEAT PASTA WITH PESTO SAUCE

This is a rather light pesto. Basil is a powerful healing plant and when used in recipes it is said to be full of prana, bringing about healing and grounding.

- 2 cups fresh basil leaves
- 3 cloves of garlic
- ½ teaspoon seas salt
- ¼ cup olive oil
- Lemon juice to taste

Combine the basil, garlic and salt in a blender and pulse to chop basil leaves. Then add olive oil slowly, blending after each addition, making a thick green paste. Add the lemon juice for flavor.
Cook whole-wheat pasta according to package direction. Drain. While hot toss with pesto sauce. Sprinkle fresh Parmesan cheeses on top and serve.

About 4 serving   188 calories per serving.

TABBOULEH

According to biblical Scholars the Bible makes reference to eating a parched grain, which was the forerunner to tabbouleh, and is still popular throughout the Middle East.

- 1-cup fine grain bulgur wheat
- 3 cups boiling water
- 1 bunch finely chopped scallions
- 2 cups chopped parsley
- 4 tablespoons of lemon juice
- ½ cup chopped radishes
- 3 tablespoons olive oil
- 1 teaspoon of sharp mustard
- Romaine lettuce leaves

Place the wheat in a large bowl or pan and pour in the boiling water. Let soak for 30 minutes or until tender. Drain the wheat and combine with other ingredients, except the lettuce leaves. Chill. Heap salad on a plate and arrange the romaine leaves around the sides so they can be used as a scoop.

Use can serve parched wheat alone as a side dish by simply adding the boiling water to the bulgur and let stand until tender and fluffy.

Chicken Dishes

CHICKEN CACCIATORE STEW

- 2 ½- 3 pounds skinless boneless chicken parts cut into small chunks
- 1 medium onion sliced
- 1 16-ounce can stew tomatoes
- 1- 8 ounce can tomato sauce
- 1 ½ teaspoon of oregano
- ½ teaspoon of minced garlic
- 1 medium green pepper sliced
- 4 medium sized carrots sliced
- 10 medium mushrooms sliced
- ¼ pound fresh whole green beans

Brown chicken in a little olive oil, in a cast iron stewing pot. Add onions, green peppers and garlic. Stir and sauté lightly. Mix together tomatoes, tomato sauce, and oregano. Pour over chicken. Add carrots, green beans and mushrooms heat to simmer for 35 minutes, stirring occasionally. Serve in bowls with toasted bread or rolls or over a bed of rice.
Makes 4 servings.

CHICKEN TOMASI

This is an adaptation from a traditional Hungarian recipe supposedly named after the town of Tomasi.

- 3 pounds of boneless, skinless chicken parts cut into bite size pieces.
- 2 teaspoons of olive oil
- 1 medium onion chopped
- 1 clove of garlic, finely chopped
- 3-5 teaspoons of paprika
- ¼ teaspoon of cayenne pepper
- ½ cup chicken broth
- 8-ounce container of nonfat plain yogurt
- ¼ cup low fat milk
- Salt and pepper to taste.

Brown chicken in olive oil. Remove to a platter and drain on a paper towel. Sauté onion and garlic in the olive oil until tender. Return chicken to pan. Sprinkle with cayenne pepper and paprika. Pour in the broth. Simmer covered until chicken is tender or about 20 minutes. Remove pan form heat. Remove chicken with slotted spoon to a platter. Keep warm. Let sauce cool to warm. Stir together in a bowl the yogurt and milk until smooth. Stir in a little of the warm sauce. Stir yogurt mixture back into saucepan. Place over low heat and add salt and pepper to taste. Return chicken to saucepan and gently reheat but do not boil. Serve over rice or couscous, or with a dinner salad and fresh bread.

Makes 6 servings, 182 calories each serving (without rice)

CURRY CHICKEN

- 2/3-cup nonfat plain yogurt
- 2 cloves of minced garlic
- 1/1/2 teaspoon of curry powder
- ¼ teaspoon of ground ginger
- Dash of cayenne pepper
- 2 pounds of boneless, skinless chicken parts cut into chunks
- ½ cup chopped fresh onion
- 1-½ cups of chopped fresh tomatoes
- 1 bay leaf
- 4 tablespoons of fresh chopped cilantro leaves

Combine yogurt and spices in medium bowl. Add chicken parts and turn to coat. Let stand at room temperature for 30 minutes. Sauté onion in a skillet with olive oil until lightly brown. Add tomatoes and bay leaf; lower heat and simmer for 5 minutes. Add chicken and yogurt mixture and stir to combine. Bring mixture back to a boil. Lower heat; cover simmer, turning once or twice until chicken is tender, about 30 minutes. Remove bay leaf and serve each serving with a topping of fresh chopped cilantro. Serve plain or over rice and vegetables.

Makes 4 servings

CHICKEN AND SCALLION MEDALLIONS

- 2 boneless, skinless chicken breasts
- 4 scallions, white part only
- ¼ cup low sodium soy sauce
- 2 tablespoons of white wine vinegar
- 2 cups of bean sprouts
- 2 cups fresh spinach leaves, rinsed with stems removed

Use a mallet to flatten the chicken breast between two pieces of wax paper. Flatten to about 1/8 inch thick. Peel off wax paper and sprinkle with salt and pepper to taste. Arrange 2 scallions across the center of each breast and roll tightly. Tie the ends of the chicken breast with kitchen string. In a bowl combine soy sauce and vinegar. Add chicken, turn to coat and marinate for 15 minutes.

In a steamer bring to boil about an inch of water. Place chicken in steamer and cook for 15 minutes, turning once. While steaming, bring marinade to a boil in small sauce pan and boil for 2 minutes.

When chicken rolls are cooked, remove from steamer, cut string and slice into ½ slices. Arrange on a bed of spinach topped with bean sprouts and pour warm marinade over the top.

Serves 2

CHICKEN IN APPLE MUSTARD SAUCE

- 4 chicken breasts boned and skinned
- 2 tablespoons of olive oil
- 1-cup organic apple juice
- 1 medium onion sliced
- 1 clove of garlic minced
- ½ teaspoon of thyme
- 4 teaspoons of Dijon mustard
- 1 apple cored and sliced

Flatten chicken with the dull side of a heavy knife. Add chicken to a skillet that has been coated with the olive oil and brown. Add the apple juice, onion, garlic and thyme. Cover and cook 10-12 minutes or until chicken is tender. Remove chicken; keep warm. Bring liquid to a boil and add mustard. Stir well. Add apple slices. Pour sauce over chicken.

Serve 4   serve with fresh steamed broccoli.

MANGO LIME CHICKEN

Rub one boneless skinless chicken breast with ½ teaspoon of chili powder. Broil and slice. Combine 1 cup diced fresh mango and 2 teaspoons each of honey, lime juice and minced scallions. Spoon over chicken. Makes one serving

CHINESE CHICKEN AND GREENS

Coat 2 boneless skinless chicken breast with a blend of 2 teaspoons each of soy sauce and oriental sesame oil. Broil. Shred chicken. Combine ¼ cup apricot jam and 1 tablespoon of hoisin sauce. Toss with chicken, and serve over lightly steamed Bok choy. Serves two about 375 calories per serving

CRANBERRY CHICKEN

Rub one boneless skinless chicken breast with crumbled rosemary. Broil. For sauce combine 1/3 cup cranberry sauce, ¼ cup chopped orange sections and 1 teaspoon minced crystallized ginger. Pour sauce over top of chicken. Serves one

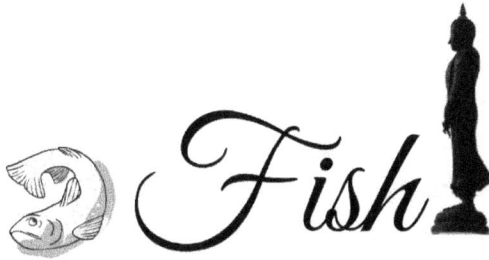

The fish recipes chosen here all supply a great source of omega 3, the essential fatty acid.

CHILLED POACHED SALMON

- 3 cups water
- 1 cup white wine
- 1 lemon sliced
- ¼ cup sliced scallions
- ¼ tsp sea salt and ¼ teaspoon black pepper
- 4-1-inch-thick salmon steaks

In large skillet, combine water, wine, lemon slices, scallions, salt and pepper. Heat to boiling and add salmon steaks and cover. Reduce heat to low. Simmer gently for 7 to 10 minutes. Remove fish from liquid. Cover and refrigerate until chilled. Makes four servings

SPICY SALMON DINNER

Poach 4 salmon fillets as above recipe. While salmon is poaching heat 1 tablespoon of olive oil and add 2 teaspoons of curry powder and sauté 15 seconds. Add sliced scallions (2 bunches – bottoms only) 2 ripe pears cored and sliced and 1 red pepper cut into julienne strips. Place warm salmon on serving plates and top with sauce and sauté vegetables and fruit.

Serves 4

SALMON TANDORI

- Juice of one lemon
- 4 salmon steaks
- 1 cup plain nonfat yogurt
- 1 (1 inch) piece of fresh ginger peeled and chopped
- 2 cloves of garlic chopped
- 1 jalapeno pepper chopped
- 1 teaspoon of black peppercorns
- 1 teaspoon of garam masala
- ½ teaspoon of turmeric
- fresh cilantro
- 4 lemons for garnish

Pour lemon juice over the salmon. Combine the yogurt, ginger, garlic, jalapeno, peppercorns, garam masala, and turmeric in a blender and blend until smooth. Spoon the mixture over the salmon and refrigerate for at least 4 hours. Preheat the oven to 500 degrees and bake the salmon for 10 minutes, until flakes easily with a fork. Garnish it with sprigs of cilantro and serve with lemon wedges.

Serves 4   259 calories

Protein 38 g carbohydrates 11g

HERBED HALIBUT

For a quick and easy main dish this recipe can't be beat. Use this topping for any fish. Try cod, haddock or salmon.

- 4 halibut fillets, about 2 pounds total
- sea salt and pepper to taste
- ¼ non-dairy, low-fat mayonnaise
- 2 tablespoons of fresh parsley

Heat the broiler. Sprinkle the halibut fillets with salt and pepper and spread the mayonnaise on top of each fillet. Put in a shallow broiler pan and broil until the fish is just opaque, 5 –10 minutes. Sprinkle the fillets with the chopped parsley before serving.

Serves 4   189 calories
Protein 32g   carbohydrates 1g

TUNA STEAK DIONNE

- 2 pounds of tuna steak cut into 4 slices
- ¼ cup whole wheat flour
- 1 teaspoon of safflower oil
- 2 tablespoons mined shallots or scallions
- 1 tablespoon of chopped capers
- 1 tablespoon minced fresh parsley
- 1 teaspoon Dijon mustard
- 1 teaspoon of Worcestershire sauce
- ¼ cup clam juice or chicken broth
- 4 medium size mushroom caps

Dredge fillets through flour. Heat safflower oil in skillet, add fish and sauté for 3 minutes on each side. Pour off oil. Heat olive oil in skillet and add shallots and capers and sauté for 1 minute. Stir in parsley, mustard, Worcestershire sauce and clam juice and cook for 2 minutes. Return fish to skillet and cook 2 minutes on each side, coating with the sauce.   Remove fish to serving plates. Add mushrooms caps to skillet and cook for 1 minute. Pour sauce over steak topping with one mushroom each. Garnish with fresh parsley.

Serves 4   calories 172

SPICY MANGO SHRIMP

Packed with beta-carotene, high in vitamin c, potassium, and fiber, a cup of mango slices contains only about 100 calories.

- 1 mango peeled
- 2 tablespoon of lemon juice
- 1-pound large shrimp peeled
- 1-tablespoon chicken stock
- 1 teaspoon of chili powder
- ¼ teaspoon of hot-pepper sauce
- 1 ½ cups canned, unsweetened crushed pineapple
- 1 cup chopped tomatoes
- 1 red onion chopped
- Mixed organic greens

Puree mango with lemon juice in a blender. In a nonstick frying pan, combine shrimp with stock, chili powder, and hot-pepper sauce, and cook, stirring, about three minutes. Mix in pineapple, tomatoes, onions, sauté until onions are tender. Spoon shrimp onto greens and drizzle with mango puree.

Serves 4   207 calories

MUSSELS STEAMED OVER TOMATOES AND BASIL

- 36 medium mussels about 2/1/2 pounds
- 3 tablespoons of olive oil
- 2 cloves of garlic, sliced and peeled
- Dash of red pepper
- ¼ cup finely shredded fresh basil
- 1 cup drained canned Italian plum tomatoes diced
- Dash of seas salt and ground black pepper

Rinse the mussels under cold water. Heat the oil in a large deep skillet over medium heat. Add the garlic and red pepper. Sauté until the garlic is tender but not brown. Stir in the basil and sauté for a few seconds. Stir in tomatoes. Simmer until tomatoes are soft, about 3 minutes. Season with salt and pepper. Add mussels, cover and heat until the mussels open, about 4 minutes. Spoon some mussels and cooking liquid into serving bowls.

Serves 6   about 71 calories

Breads

Bread is considered the "staff of life." Every culture has some form of bread that is served with a meal.

PEANUT BUTTER BREAD

- 1-cup whole whet flour
- ½ cup corn meal
- ½ cup oatmeal
- 2 teaspoons of baking powder
- ½ teaspoon of cinnamon
- Mix together in a bowl.
- Add;
- 1 packet of stevia
- ½ cup peanut butter
- 1 egg
- 1 teaspoon of olive oil
- 2 tablespoons of nonfat plain yogurt
- 1-cup water.

Mix until well blended. Pour into a nonstick (or lightly sprayed) 4x8 inch loaf pan. Bake at 30 minutes, until lightly brown. Remove to cooling rack. Slice to serve. Serve plain or topped with honey or jam. Toast lightly and top with honey or jam for breakfast.

Serves 8   149 calories

BEER BREAD

- 2 cups of whole-wheat flour
- ¼ cup rye flour
- 2-1/4 teaspoons of double acting baking powder
- 1 teaspoon of seas salt
- 3 packets of stevia
- 1 –12 ounce can beer at room temperature

Preheat over to 375 degrees.

In large bowl, sift flour, baking powder, salt and stevia. Add beer. Stir until foam subsides and all ingredients are moistened. Place dough in a 4x8 inch loaf pan that has been sprayed with a nonstick cooking spray. (Dough will be loose). Bake 45-59 minutes, until golden brown. Cool bread in pan for 5 minutes. Then remove to a rack to finish cooling.

For a variation add 1-teaspoon caraway seeds with beer.

Serves 12   93 calories

Protein 3g   carbohydrates 20g

FRUIT BREADS

These can be used as a dessert or as breakfast bread.

BLUEBERRY LEMON BREAD

- 2 tablespoons of olive oil
- 2 egg whites
- 1 tablespoon of nonfat plain yogurt
- 2 cups of soy flour or whole-wheat flour
- 1 ½ teaspoon baking powder
- ½ teaspoon of baking soda
- 2 tablespoons of lemon juice
- 1-cup blueberries
- ½ cup water
- 3 packets of stevia

Mix olive oil, yogurt, and egg whites. Add other ingredients and mix well. Pour into a 9x5 loaf pan that has been sprayed with a non-stick cooking spray. Bake at 350 degrees for 35-45 minutes or until done. Remove to cooling rack and let cool.

Options – add chopped nuts if desired.

ORANGE RAISIN BREAD

- ¼ cup boiling water
- ½ cup raisins
- 1 small orange
- 4 packets of stevia
- 1 egg white
- 1 teaspoon of vanilla extract

- 2 ½ teaspoons of olive oil
- 1/2-cup whole wheat plus ½- soy flour
- ½ teaspoon baking powder
- ½ teaspoon baking soda
- 1/8-teaspoon sea salt
- ½ teaspoon ground cinnamon
- ¼ teaspoon ground nutmeg
- ¼ teaspoon ground ginger

Preheat oven 325 degree. Pour boiling water over raisins in a small bowl and set aside. Grate the rind of the orange. Peel off any rind left on the orange and cut the orange into pulp. Place the orange pulp, raisins and water into a blender and blend until raisins are chopped but not puree. In a large bowl, combine raisin mixture, orange rind, stevia, egg white, vanilla, and oil. Mix with a spoon. Sift the flour, baking powder and baking soda, salt and spices together. Add to wet ingredients and stir to moisten. Place batter in a 4x8 inch nonstick loaf pan, sprayed with a non-stick cooking spray. Bake for 35 minutes, until lightly browned. Cool in pan for 10 minutes and then remove to rack for cooling.

Serves 5   169 calories
Protein 4g   Carbohydrates   34g

Options – add chopped walnuts or almonds

CRANBERRY-NUT BREAD

- 1-½ tablespoons wheat germ
- 1 orange
- 2/3 cup unsweetened apple juice
- 4 ounces of tofu
- ¼ cup safflower oil
- 1/3-cup orange blossom honey or other mild honey
- 1-cup whole-wheat flour and 1 cup of soy flour
- ½ teaspoon of sea salt
- 1 teaspoon of baking soda
- 1 teaspoon of baking powder
- 1 cup fresh cranberries rinsed
- ½ cup lightly toasted walnuts or pecans coarsely chopped

Preheat over to 350 degrees. Grease 8 1/2 x 4 ½ loaf pan with a non sticking cooking spray. Dust with wheat germ. Finely grate orange zest into a medium-size bowl. Juice orange and add enough apple juice to equal 1 cup. In a blender, blend the tofu and a small amount of juice. With blender running, gradually add remaining juice; blend until smooth. Whisk honey, oil and orange zest. In another bowl, sift next four ingredients; add to wet mixture and stir gently until batter forms. Fold in cranberries and nuts. Spread batter in pan and bake for 50-60 minutes, until bread is well browned and done. Cool in pan for 10 minutes and turn onto a cooling rack.

Serves 8   145 calories

EZEKIEL'S BREAD

This recipe is one of the few specific recipes found in the Bible. Neither Ezekiel nor the people who made and ate the bread realized that they were practicing what is known as 'augmentation'. It means to pack highly potent grains and quality protein into bread rather than eat bread made of one grain. This bread adds beans to the recipe to give it protein. According to the Bible the people of the middle East ate a wide range of beans. Ezekiel's bread is a good source of protein, calcium, phosphorous, iron, potassium, vitamin A and C, thiamin, riboflavin and niacin.

- 2 packets of yeast
- ½ cup warm water
- 4 cups whole-wheat flour
- 2 1/4 cups barley flour
- 1-cup soy flour
- ¼ cup rye flour
- 1/3 cup of honey
- ½ cup cooked and mashed chick peas or lentil beans
- 4 tablespoons olive oil
- 2 cups water
- ½ tablespoon seas salt

Dissolve yeast in warm water with 1 tablespoon of honey. Set aside for 10 minutes. Combine the next five ingredients. Blend lentils or chick peas, oil, remaining honey, and a small amount of water in a blender and blend. Place in a large bowl with remaining water. Stir in 1 cup of the mixed flour. Add the yeast mixture. Stir in salt and remaining flour. Place on floured bread board and knead until smooth. Put in oiled bowl and let rise until doubled in bulk. Knead again, cut dough and shape into two loaves. Place in greased pans and let rise. Bake at 375 degrees for 45 minutes to 1hour.

Note; there is a reference in the passage to adding 'fitches', which is a seasoning or herb. It has been suggested that the herbs are cumin, fennel and nutmeg. If you wish add 1 teaspoon of cumin, fennel or nutmeg.

Desserts

BAKED APPLES WITH RAISINS

- 4 large baking apples
- 2 tablespoons of raisins
- ½ teaspoon of cinnamon and ½ teaspoon of nutmeg
- ¼ cup of unsweetened apple juice
- 1 packet of stevia

Core apples. Remove a strip of peel from the top of each apple. Cut a slice off the bottom of each apple, so the apples sit flat. Toss raisins, cinnamon, nutmeg and stevia. Fill each apple with some of the spiced raisins. Place apples in a shallow baking dish and pour the apple juice around the apples. Cover and bake for 30 minutes in 400-degree preheated oven.
Serve warm or chill.

Variations- Preheat oven to 450 degrees. Best 2 egg whites with ¼ teaspoon of crème of tartar and 3 packets of stevia until soft peaks form. Place apples on a non-stick cooking sheet. Top with meringue and bake for 5 minutes until just brown.
With meringue about 75 calories each

Serves 4

HONEY CAKE

Serving honey is an ancient way of honoring guest. Honey was served after the main meal and at the end of the day because it has a claming and tranquilizing effect.

* 1-cup honey
* ½ cup melted butter or ½ cup almond oil
* 1teaspoon of cinnamon
* ½ teaspoon of seas salt
* ½ cup milk
* 3 eggs
* 4-cups - whole-wheat flour.

Cream together the butter or oil and honey. Add eggs. Sift dry ingredients together and add to creamed mixture alternately with the milk. Pour the batter into two oiled 9-inch cake pans. Bake for 35 minutes in oven preheated to 350 degrees.
Variation – place the batter into one glass oiled cake pan.

BANANA ICE CREAM

Bananas are one of nature's perfect foods. This recipe uses frozen bananas to create an ice cream like dessert without all the fat and sugar.

Freeze bananas in the peel. Run under warm water and peel the banana when you want to use them. This will keep the bananas from turning brown. Do not remove the stringy part as this is full of nutrients and will blend right in.

In a blender or food processor place two frozen, peeled and cut up in chunks bananas. Add 2 tablespoons of kefir.   Add two large strawberries halved and 4-5 blackberries or blueberries, Add 1 tablespoon of warm water. Blend until thick and smooth
Mix in chopped pecans, almonds or walnuts if desired.

LAYERED FRUIT SALAD

Needed to serve 8

* 1 pound of red grapes
* 2 bananas
* 2 fresh sliced peaches
* 1-pint fresh raspberries
* 2 oranges
* 3 kiwis
* Juice from 2 oranges
* 4 packets of stevia – optional

Rinse grapes. Cut in half and remove seeds. Place in bottom of glass serving bowl. Peel and slice bananas. Place over grapes. Slice peaches and place on top of bananas. Rinse raspberries and sprinkle on top of peaches. Peel oranges and cut into small pieces.   Place on top of raspberries. Peel and slice kiwis and place on top of salad.   Pour orange juice over the top of salad and sprinkle with stevia. Keep salad refrigerator until ready to eat.

137 calories

Protein 2g carbohydrates 33g

CARROT CAKE

- 1 ½ cups whole-wheat flour
- 1 teaspoon each of baking powder and baking soda
- 1 ½ teaspoon of ground cinnamon
- ½ teaspoon of nutmeg
- 8 packets of stevia
- 2 tablespoons plus 2 teaspoons of olive oil
- 2 eggs
- 2 egg whites
- 1 teaspoon of vanilla
- 1 cup unsweetened crushed canned pineapple
- ¼ cup liquid drained form pineapple
- 1 cup finely shredded carrots
- ¼ cup raisins

Preheat oven to 350 degrees. In a small bowl combine dry ingredients. In a large bowl combine sweetener, oil, eggs, vanilla and pineapple liquid. Beat at low speed with an electric beater until smooth. Add dry ingredients and beat until just moistened. Stir in pineapple, carrots, and rinsing, mixing well. Spoon mixture into 8 inch square baking pan that has been sprayed with a nonstick cooking spray. Bake 20-25 minutes. Cool in pan. Remove and serve plain or frost.

FROSTING

- 1-cup ricotta cheese
- 1-teaspoon vanilla
- 3 packets of stevia

Combine all ingredients and beat until smooth. Spread over the top of the cake.

Serves 8   256 calories with frosting

Protein 10g   carbohydrates 30g

OATMEAL PIE CRUST

Use this piecrust for cheesecake recipe as well as fruit pie recipes.

- 1-cup whole-wheat flour
- ½ cup rolled oats
- ¼ cup olive oil
- 2 tablespoons of water

Please the flour and oats in a nine-inch pie pan and mix well. Slowly stir in the oil. Mix with a fork to evenly distribute the oil. Gradually stir in enough water to make mixture hold together when pressed. Press the dough against the sides and bottom of the pie pan. Poke some small holes in the bottom of the crust to keep it from puffing up. Bake at 375 degrees for 20 minutes or until the crust is light brown.

Variations - add 1 teaspoon of cinnamon to flour-oat mixture.

FRUIT TOPPED TOFU CHEESECAKE

Prepare 1 unbaked oatmeal piecrust

- 1 teaspoon of cinnamon
- 1 cup mashed tofu
- 1 cup chopped almonds
- ½ cup honey
- 1 cup soymilk
- 1 ½ tablespoon arrowroot
- 1 ½ teaspoons of vanilla
- 2 teaspoons of lemon juice
- 2 teaspoons grated lemon rind

Place nuts, tofu, honey, soymilk, arrowroot, vanilla, lemon juice and grated lemon rind in food processor and blend until smooth. Pour into three unbaked piecrusts. Bake at 350 degrees for 30 minutes or until set. Chill. When pie is thoroughly chilled arrange 1 ½ cups of sliced strawberries, blueberries or any other berry you choose over the top of the pie. Place the remaining ½ cup of berries in a saucepan with ¼ cup water and 3 tablespoons of honey and 1 tablespoon of cornstarch. Bring to a boil. L Lower heat and simmer until cornstarch is dissolved and sauce starts to thicken (about 5 minutes). Let cool to room temperature and then pour over the top of cheesecake.
Makes 1- 9-inch cheesecake.

WORLD'S BEST STRAWBERRY PIE

This is the only recipe in this book that contains sugar. This is such a great pie that I thought I would include it in this book. Use organic raw sugar.

1 baked oatmeal piecrust.
4 cups hulled, washed strawberries
¾ cup water
¾ cup organic sugar – Wholesome Sweeteners
3 tablespoons of cornstarch
¼ teaspoon sea salt
Place 3 cups of whole fresh strawberries into baked piecrust and set aside.

Crush one-cup strawberries in small saucepan; add water, bring to a boil, simmer for 3 minutes. Strain juice from cooked strawberries and add water if needed to make one cup of liquid.
Combine sugar, cornstarch and salt in same small saucepan; slowly add strawberry juice, stirring until smooth. Bring to boil, stirring constantly; cook 3 minutes until thick and clear.; remove from heat.

Spoon glaze over the 3 cups of strawberries that have been arranged in the piecrust. Be careful to coat each berry. Chill pie for several hours. Serve for a rich dessert serve with whipped cream or ice cream.

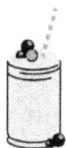 Yogi Drinks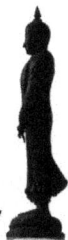

Yogi drinks help to cleanse and revitalize the body. The yogi vitality drink is used to both cleanse the internal system and to act as a tonic to tonify or build up the energy of the system.

Add the juice of ½ lemon and 1-3 teaspoons of blackstrap molasses to 8 ounces of hot water. A little honey may be added for flavor. The lemon juice helps to cleanse the body of phlegm and waste and the molasses helps the body to increase its iron and mineral intake. It is recommended that the yogi drink be taken every 3rd or 5th night for several weeks and then only when needed thereafter for strength and cleansing.

GINGER TEA

Ginger tea is both calming to the nerves and energizing to the body. Ginger is a great digestive aid that is good for every body. It is especially good for women during their monthly menses.

• 4-6 1/8-inch-thick slices of fresh ginger root
• 2 cups water
• 1 tablespoon lemon juice and 1 teaspoon of honey.

Bring water to a boil and add ginger root slices. Boil until water is lightly brown in color. Remove from heat. Add fresh lemon juice and honey. Pour and serve.

YOGI TEA

This healthy tea is a great substitute for coffee. Anna-maya-kosha-yoga (the science of yogic food) teaches that the spices included in this tea have the following properties:

-
- Cardamom pods – digestive aid
- Ginger root – healing for colds and flue – increases energy
- Black pepper – a blood purifier
- Cloves – nervous system
- Cinnamon- strengthens the bones

The milk in the tea helps with the assimilation of the spices. Add a pinch of black tea to alloy the ingredients and create the right chemical balance.

To 2 quarts of water add:
- Whole cloves – 15
- Cardamom pods – 16
- Cinnamon – 5- 2-inch sticks
- Ginger root – 8 slices

Boil gently for 30 - 40 minutes (adding water if it evaporates), then add:
- ½ teaspoon black tea
- 3-4 cups of milk

Bring to a boil. Turn off heat and add honey to taste. Makes 2-3 quarts. Can be stored in the refrigerator for up to a week with the milk added.

Mango Lassi

A lassi is a yogurt-based drink, excellent for breakfast or as a snack. Mangos are recommended for live disorders, menstrual problems and general digestive disorders. Yogurt is recommended for its beneficial bacteria. When combined together this drink makes an excellent tonic for the entire digestive system.

- 2 cups plain nonfat yogurt
- 2 medium very ripe mangos peeled and sliced
- 2-3 tablespoons of maple syrup or honey
- 6 ice cubes or 2/3 cups water
- ¼ teaspoon or rosewater – optional

Blend at high speed until smooth and creamy. Makes approximately 4 cups.

Sesame – Ginger Milk

This drink is nourishing to the nervous system and is said to be healthful for the make sexual organs, stimulating the production of healthy sexual fluids.

- ¼ cup sesame seeds
- 2 tablespoons coarsely chopped fresh peeled ginger root
- 12 ounces of milk
- 2 teaspoons of honey or maple syrup

Blend at high sped until smooth and frothy. Makes 2 cups.

SANGRIA

By now we all know that red wine is a great source of antioxidants. Again, remember everything in moderation.

- 2 oranges cut in wedges
- 2 lemons cut in wedges
- 1 fifth - of red wine
- 2 packets of stevia
- 2 tablespoons of brandy
- 1 apple cored and cut in wedges
- 1 12-ounce bottle of sparkling water

Thread fruit on a long skewer. Place the wine, stevia and brandy in a large pitcher. Place fruit in the pitch and let marinate by chilling for 1 hour. Add sparkling water to the pitcher and serve into individual glasses.

Substitute organic grape juice for wine if you prefer to not drink alcohol and omit brandy.

Anna Mayer Kosha Yoga reminds us that yoga is all inclusive.
Nothing goes unnoticed, and that includes,
what and how we eat!

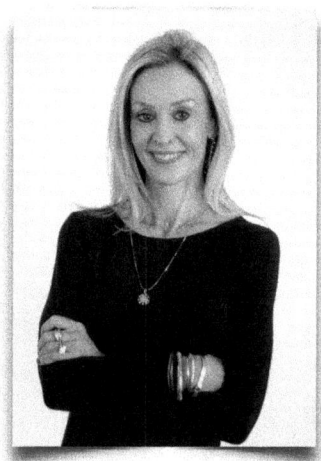

ABOUT THE AUTHOR

Born on a small island off the coast of Maine, Doctor Lynn grew up in a small village where folk medicine was routinely practiced. She left the island as a young single mother on welfare to enter college at the University of Maine. She graduated with a degree in Communication and then went on to study Naturopathy, Aromatherapy, Herbology, Yoga therapy and Fitness affiliation with ACE.

She has over 30 years' of experience in teaching, writing and producing books and videos on how to stay healthy, happy, find wealth and discover Inner wisdom of your body, mind and soul. Her inspiring life journey from her humble beginnings to a wealthy world traveler, published author, international speaker, TV and DVD producer, Doctor Lynn will share with you what it takes to live a healthy, wealthy, happy and peaceful life in your body, mind and soul.

Doctor Lynn lives in Sarasota, Florida with her husband Dan. She is the mother of two children; Derek and Kristen, and the grandmother of three; Gareth, Sam and Mia who give her the greatest joy in life.

Visit the author online at:
DoctorLynn.com